SOCIAL EVOLUTION OF LOVE

Dedicated to my late teacher and friend Miss O Wai-sheung

Social Evolution of Love

A study of mate selection among psychiatric sufferers

MARCUS Y.L. CHIU
Department of Social Work
Hong Kong Baptist University

Routledge
Taylor & Francis Group
LONDON AND NEW YORK

First published 1999 by Ashgate Publishing

Reissued 2018 by Routledge
2 Park Square, Milton Park, Abingdon, Oxon OX14 4RN
52 Vanderbilt Avenue, New York, NY 10017

Routledge is an imprint of the Taylor & Francis Group, an informa business

A Library of Congress record exists under LC control number: 99072557

ISBN 13: 978-1-138-34789-2 (hbk)
ISBN 13: 978-0-429-43682-6 (ebk)

Contents

List of Tables and Figures

Acknowledgements

This book has originated from my doctoral research work at The University of Manchester. Among many individuals who have offered invaluable help and support throughout the process of completing this book, my first gratitude and respect go to Professor Peter Huxley who was my research supervisor. He has provided his guidance, encouragement, and thoughtful comments throughout this research study, and at critical points. His comments are often short, sharp and articulate enough to pull me out from muddling ideas.

I would to thank the patients and their spouses who were willing to take part in this study. I must also thank Professor Creed, Dr. Bridges, Dr. McGrath, and Dr. Procter of Department of Psychiatry, M.R.I. for their support and allowing me to contact their patients. Mr. David Lyne and his secretary at Making Space were also very helpful in contacting their members for this study. I have several discussions with Dr. Tsui Kai-wing of the Chinese University of Hong Kong. His expertise on human genetics has enriched my view on the wonders and difficulties in this specialised area. Professor Robert Harris is visiting the department and he has given valuable opinions for the part on genetics and ethics.

I owed my wife for her understanding, patience and kindness in excusing me from many family occasions because of this work. Finally I want to thank my late but dear teacher and friend Miss O Wai-sheung. Without her encouragement and advice, I would not have gone to England for further studies.

Readers may find mistakes and deficiencies when they go through this book. It remains strictly a matter of my own responsibility for the shortfalls.

Introduction

Mate selection has long been a concern for academics of various disciplines like geneticists, anthropologists, social psychologists, and sociologists. In the normal population, there is ample evidence that propinquity, physical attractiveness, and situational feelings are closely linked with initial liking. Married couples are found to be significantly and positively correlated in age, height (Susane & Lepage, 1988), weight (Schafer & Keith, 1990), socio-economic status, intelligence quotient, certain psychological traits (Vandenberg, 1972; Eysenck, 1975; Watkin & Meredith, 1981; Mascie-Taylor, 1987, 1988; Mascie-Taylor & Vandenberg, 1988; Gilger, 1991), and even surnames (Lasker, 1968, 1985). Nicholson (1992) compared five major similarity studies that used the clinical scales of Minnesota Personality Inventory (MMPI) in the period 1965 – 1985. Significant, but different within-couple similarity was found and there was no recognizable and generalized pattern.

Spouse similarity can be explained in alternative ways (Price & Vandenberg, 1980). First, initial liking – for some reasons, people are drawn to choose a partner who is similar to them in certain ways. It is this concern that interests academics because of its implication on the genetic structure of the population (Crow & Felsenstein, 1968; Freire-Maia, 1968; Plomin et al, 1990). Second, convergence – interpersonal interaction through living together has either eroded the difference or increased the similarity. The similarity observed is but a result sampling bias because dissimilar couples like those who are separated or divorced are not picked up. Fourth, the similarity is just a function of age. People usually choose a partner in the same age group, making the within-couple correlation high. Accordingly, the similarity, as indicated by significant correlation, is indeed a manifestation of co-variation between the age of the couple rather than the dimension that it intends to measure. Most studies on spouse similarity among normal population are cross-sectional, owing to the many practical obstacles of obtaining longitudinal data. The similarity data continued to be used as a parameter estimate for genetic and environmental influence in the belief that there is an initial assortment between the couple.

Only recently, this belief has been supported with longitudinal findings. Feng and Baker (1994) surveyed at three different time points (i.e. 1971/72, 1984/85, 1988) altogether almost nine hundred couples in the areas of attitudes, personality traits and psychological well-being. With the use of multiple regression, they were able to remove the effect of intervening factors like age and education and observed the changes over reasonable time length. They found that spouse correlation were high for attitudes and low to moderate for personality and psychological well-being. The pure-effect correlations did not change considerably over time and this held true even when subjects were regrouped according to the length of marriage. The findings indicated that age covariation or educational background affected very little the similarities, and that couples in fact diverged, not converged over time.

On one hand, these similarity or assortment factors can be explained by the availability and constraints imposed by class stratification and the resultant differential access to social and economic resources. Social homogamy (similarity in social characteristics) between spouses can be seen essentially as a function of social stratification, and serves in turn the function of preserving the cultural, social and economic resources of its own class. On the other hand, evolutionists consider mate selection functional for reproduction and adaptation. Women tend to prefer a spouse with reproductive advantages (better resources for the nurture of fertility and offspring), while men's preferences are based more on the indirect observation of reproductive capacity (i.e. physical attractiveness, and domestic ability). Finally current family studies suggested a more social and dynamic view of how people create a social environment that facilitates and rein-forces one's own psychological attributes by selecting a mate with similar or compatible disposition or traits.

Whatever the interpretation, it is clear that mate selection is not a random process. People tend to choose partners who are geographically near, of similar socio-economically background, having similar psychological traits, and from the same culture (Epstein & Guttman, 1984). Personal preference plays an important role in the selection of a mate and there is a sex difference with regard to these preferences. Men favour physically attractive and domestically capable partners more than women do for their partners, while women favour more than men do a partner with secure economic resources (Buss & Barnes, 1986; Buss, 1989). Similarity between spouses is found in physical traits, psychological and cognitive traits, religiosity, and activity level (Macie-Taylor, 1987; 1988). These similarities may have social and genetic implications.

Assortment has been found among certain groups. Barlow and colleagues (1997) surveyed 5878 attenders of a sexually transmitted disease clinic in London over a period of about three years and found the sexual mixing of the subjects highly assortative. Although it is widely accepted that cardiovascular risk increased with age and environmental factors like eating habit and life style, which is very much affected or shared by one's partner, health survey among spouses did not indicated consistent increase with marriage duration (Knuiman et al, 1996). Therefore, it has been suggested that assortment of certain disposition to the risks factor may be a more plausible explanation.

Far less is known about psychiatric patients in these respects than about the normal population. Patients and their spouses have been found to be of low social background (Becker, 1963; Alanen & Kinnunen, 1975), but it is not certain whether this is a consequence of the illness (downward-drift) (Kohn, 1968), accumulated premorbid social disadvantages, or homogamy of backgrounds between the families. In the literature there is most interest in the similarity of diagnosis and symptomatology in couples, one or both of whom are ill. Knowledge of mate selection among psychotic patients from other points of view is virtually non-existent.

Various studies have been conducted on in-patient populations (Penrose, 1944; Slater & Woodside, 1951; Gregory, 1959; Kreitman, 1968), out-patient populations (Kreitman, 1962, 1964; Nielsen, 1964; Hare & Shaw, 1965; Pond et al, 1963; Agulnik, 1970; Ovenstone, 1973), and community samples (Buck & Ladd, 1965; Hagnell & Kreitman, 1974). In general, they have found a greater than chance excess of spouses both having been ill, and / or having the same diagnosis or similar symptomatology. In spite of different hypotheses about the causes of this situation, most authors suggested that assortment of a certain kind has taken place between the couples, one or both of whom have been referred for psychiatric services. The hypothesis that the spouse (particularly the wife) developed similar symptomatology in reaction to an ill partner has received little support, but there is some evidence that spouses of certain neurotic groups are more likely to have affected their partners than spouses of the psychotic group. Assortment of symptomatology and certain personality traits still exist after the length of marriage is controlled. This led the researchers to believe that there was an initial assortment not due to the marital interaction. The initial assortment could have happened in various ways, but may include the assortment of predisposing factors such as personality traits which may make people vulnerable to the development of certain mental disorders.

Most of these studies are cross-sectional and retrospective, because longitudinal study is more costly, and sometimes difficult if the patient population is a mobile one. These studies had the overriding clinical focus of whether the spouse of patients "has" or "has not" similar symptoms and diagnosis. Selection of partner has been treated as one discrete event rather than a developmental process (acquaintance, courtship, and marriage / living together).

The need for research into the psychosocial aspects of mate selection among psychiatric patients is well justified by its potential contribution to our greater understanding of genetic transmission, and the effect of interpersonal contexts on the causes and courses of mental disorders. While human behaviour can be genetically influenced or determined, it is equally possible that the situations leading to a particular genetic consequences can be non-genetic (e.g. psychosocial elements) in nature. If choosing a partner involves the matching of similar phenotype and that phenotype is determined genetically, this could mean a concentration of phenotypic traits in the population. If assortment also happens to the genotype, this will have a direct implication for the frequency and distribution of affected genes. In either case, the study of mate selection among patient groups would facilitate a better appreciation of the interplay of social and genetic factors.

There are four chapters of the literature review which follow this introduction. In chapter one, concordance studies among patient samples will be reviewed. It will be of interest to examine the basis for the assertion that like is choosing like. Problems with regard to differences in methodology, sampling frame and operational definitions will be discussed. In chapter two, the psychological and sociological perspectives of mate selection will be discussed. In chapter three, both the population genetics and molecular genetics of mental illness will be reviewed alongside with the recent development of evolutionist views on social adaptation and human reproductive strategy. In chapter four, ethical issues in relation to mental illness in general, and genetic improvement in particular will be discussed to reveal the complexity of the problems.

There are other aspects of non-random mate selection that are not included in the literature review. Arranged marriage is an example. The reason for its exclusion is because the practice of arranged marriage is rare today among mainstream industralised societies. Only two cases out of the fifty patients are of ethnic background (one Pakistani and one Persian), and they both did not report themselves as a case of arranged marriage. The concept of marriage or partnership to be covered in the review is also a Western and Christian one, restricting to one-to-one heterosexual relationship (monogamy). The choice for monogamous focus of this study is mainly because of the availability of information. It will be seen later the enormous difficulties in finding sufficient number of cases who are still in the marriages. Partnership of other forms are expected to be of very small proportion among treated patients, and are usually "hidden" because of the social stigma attached to it, thus making them difficult to be identified.

Although same-sex partnership in general population has increasingly drawn much academic interest recently (Buss & Schmitt, 1993; Bailey et al, 1994; Kenrick et al, 1990,1993,1995; Huston & Schwartz, 1995), it is quite a separate theme for further investigation. Above all, possibly the greatest enthusiasm will end up in just a few cases. For this reason, partnership of the same sex, polygyny ("many wives"), and polyandry ("many husbands") are all beyond the scope of this study and the following chapters of literature review.

1 Mental Illness among Spouses of Psychiatric Patients

Concordance Studies

The initial interest to explore whether people with psychiatric problems would have spouses with similar psychiatric problems started with a series of concordance studies. The spouses of diagnosed group are also checked against diagnostic criteria to see if they are also ill or having the same diagnosis. The percentage of incidents of ill spouses can then be tabulated and compared with the expected percentage of the existing distribution. In the in-patient population, Penrose (1944) found twenty-two pairs of husbands and wives both admitted into hospital over a 34-year period. The concordance between the spouses was 36% while the observed number of cases was nine times the expected. Gregory (1959) replicated the study in Britain and had a very close estimate of excess (8.8 times) but with a much higher (64%) concordance rate. Kreitman (1968) in the South-East counties of Britain managed to find 74 pairs of in-patients whose concordance rate fell between the previous two studies (42%).

With regard to the out-patients population, Kreitman (1962) found a 1.5 times excess of observed cases and a 29% concordance in Chichester. Nielsen (1964), using a Danish sample, found very close excess (1.4) of observed cases but a slightly higher concordance (38%).

There were only two studies that used a community sample. Buck and Ladd (1965) accessed insurance records which covered about half of the Ontario population and found significantly more than expected psychoneurosis among the marital partners of patients. The other study was Hagnell and Kreitman's survey of the entire population of a district in South Sweden (1974) which arrived at an exactly the same estimate of 1.4 times excess in observed cases. They confirmed that wives were more susceptible than husbands to illness, and showed a progressive increase in morbidity with increasing duration of marriage.

The estimates obviously vary greatly from 29% to 64%. In-patient groups generally yield a higher estimate than out-patient groups. It is reasonable to believe that in-patient groups are distinct from out-patients and the general population in the community. Admission to hospital for psychiatric cases is essentially a selective process and only some of the out-patients constitute part of the in-patient population (Goldberg & Huxley, 1980). In calculating such an estimate, the total population of the targeted area must be referred to. Yet the demographic features, availability and accessibility of the psychiatric services of a particular district can be so different from others that straight-forward comparison may not be actually comparing like with like. This is particularly the case in Britain where regional differences are so marked. Unless national data has been compared and the figures adjusted, spatial variations could result in the existing differences of concordance estimates. We cannot simply assume demographic similarities either in different parts of a country or across different countries.

The only sensible conclusive remark so far from these studies is that there are more than the expected number of pairs coming for psychiatric service, and a considerable diagnostic concordance between these couples. One may argue that this phenomenon still indicates a higher occurrence of being ill and having an ill spouse than would be of random chance. Nielsen (1964) analysed twenty nine concordant pairs of new psychiatric referrals with reference to each of the five possibilities that could have resulted in concordance :

1 That the husband and wife living together tend to influence one another and that one partner may "infect" the other with abnormal reactions.
2 That similarity of environment, diet, economic state, and common sources of anxiety may contribute to common breakdown.
3 That there is a tendency for people of a similar constitution to marry each other.
4 That the illness of one partner represents a reaction to the breakdown of the other.
5 That psychiatric treatment is facilitated for the second spouse when the first to fall ill has already been in contact with psychiatric service.

He found condition (2) received least support, and that cases in his study fell into the other four possibilities or a combination of them (in depressive cases). Studies that followed attempted to answer the question whether it was the initial pattern of mating, or interaction after marriage, that accounted for the diagnostic concordance. A number of studies of patient's spouses provided more information about the symptoms, social and psychological variables of the patient (treated or untreated) and the spouse. Very often, a control group was used to ensure that significance was specific to the patient group only. These studies are reviewed next.

Slater and Woodside (1951) compared one hundred couples whose husbands were in-patient neurotics with 100 control pairs whose husbands were in-patients of a medical or a surgical ward. Significantly more wives of the probands were found to be neurotic and psychotic than the wives of the control group. In couples who were both ill, IQ, nervous predisposition and temperament were found to be positively correlated though not to a significant level. They suggested that this was due to primary assortative elements among spouses with psychiatric problems but this view was challenged by Kreitman (1964) who found initial assortment of psychological traits in a non-patient control group, but very low or even zero correlation among the patient group. In a later study Kreitman (1968) refined his argument and suggested that while initial assortative mating may happen in psychotic patients, an interactionist perspective could best explain the neurotic concordance. Kreitman (1968) also demonstrated how the failure to consider length of marriage as a decisive variable would have led to a blurred picture and probably a misleading conclusion of overall assortative mating. The Birmingham study by Pond and colleagues (1963) found a strong association between marital adjustment and neuroticism in the women of a working-class population. The authors explained the neurotic incidence in terms of the effects of present and past marital relationships and suggested that genetic predisposition plays a relatively small role.

The interactionist view of the neurotic disorders was partially supported by Ovenstone (1973) who found significant correlation in the aspect of muscle and nervous tension but not in symptomatology between the spouses. Bhagat's study (1976) on fifty attempted suicide cases and their spouses found similar personality characteristics between women who attempted suicide and their husband, but not between men who attempted suicide and their wives. It was further found that wives of male patients were distinguished in personality items from wives of a sample of normal controls, with the use of discriminant analysis. The hypotheses derived from the study were basically interactionist in nature, drawing attention to the interpersonal situation that led to the suicide.

Agulnik (1970) interviewed 40 male phobic out-patients and their spouses. He showed quite different results from previous studies that spouses of phobic patients were not demonstrably neurotic, and that neurotic manifestations in the spouse did not progressively develop with increasing duration of marriage. He suggested a stress-reaction perspective which tries to explain the differential development of symptoms of the spouse in response to the ill partner. This seemed to be in line with Hagnell and Kreitman (1974) who found that remission of illness in husbands had a clear relationship with a lower illness rating in wives (except in the lowest social class). A one-year follow-up study of 33 agoraphobic women and their husbands (Hafner, 1977) showed that a proportion of husbands were adversely affected by wives' initial symptoms, but improved when their wives showed signs of relapse.

Although the interactionist view seemed to have enlisted more support than that of initial assortment, the two approaches need not be mutually exclusive. If a genuine element of initial assortative mating exists in which people with illness or a predisposition to illness, tend to marry people with similar disposition to illness, then marital interaction can still determine the course of symptom development and remission of illness. It is self-evident that interactionist analysis of patients is only possible in those cases where some initial assortment has already happened.

It is apparent that the existing picture is far from clear, and that there is wide disagreement and differences with regard to the definition of caseness, the illness categories that are included in the study, and the operational instrument used for the indication of psychological traits and symptoms. Some authors used in-patient samples (Slater & Woodside, 1951; Kreitman, 1968) while others used out-patient samples (Kreitman, 1964; Nielsen, 1964; Agulnik, 1970; Ovenstone, 1973; Hafner, 1977) or community samples (Nielsen, 1964; Hagnell & Kreitman, 1974). Hare and Shaw had a strict criteria of a couple with at least one child under sixteen, while most others had no such specification. Some concerned spouses of both male and female patients (Kreitman, 1964, 1968; Agulnik, 1970; Bhagat, 1976) whereas some were concerned only with wives of male patients (Slater & Woodside, 1951) or husbands of female patients (Hafner, 1977). Some studies included organic psychosis, alcoholism, personality disorder, and psychopathy while others either excluded organic cases or included only a particular diagnostic group.

Conclusion

Findings of concordance studies do not seem to have moved very far beyond the initial position of suggesting a greater-than-expected frequency of diagnostic or symptomatological concordance, and the importance of the spouse on the course of illness and rehabilitation. Prolonged marital interaction with a neurotic patient sometimes makes the spouse ill, but it may well be argued that the environmental influence which the patient is under is also shared by the spouse. It could be the total environment, not just the patients that make the spouses sick. As far as the psychotic patients and their spouses are concerned, it is generally believed that the similarity in mental health and symptomatology is due to an initial assortment rather than an interaction effect. How this initial assortment happened is largely unexplained by these particular studies.

2 Psychological and Sociological Perspectives

The formation and dissolution of heterosexual partnership vary according to culture and has a history as early as mankind. While historical studies (Macfarlane, 1978; Houlbrooke, 1984; Mattinson et al, 1988) revealed how these forms of partnership changed or remained intact over time, anthropologists (Fox, 1975) studied how this biological universality was modified by culture and ecology. Psychologists pondered at the innate ability to bond and attach and subsequent development of personality (Bowlby, 1969). These attempts can be regarded as alternative interpretation of the biological forces, and at most could only explain why people need to meet someone else and to form into confiding relationship. It gives no account why one chose a particular one. In this chapter, we will visit some of the major theories from both the psychological and sociological perspectives, and we shall soon notice the complexity of the issue is beyond the coping of a single paradigm.

Psychological Perspectives

Psychoanalytic View of Parental Influence

Psychoanalyts were the first ones to concern the impact of parents on the children's choice of partner. Classical theorists described the dynamic situation between the parents and the child as Oedipal complex (Freud, 1923) and Electra complex (Jung, 1953) in which a child would have sexual impulses towards the parent of the opposite sex, and would be hostile unconsciously towards the parent of the same sex. The conflict was said to be resolved through the identification with the same-sex parent and later on through looking for a partner who is like the opposite-sex parent.

To prove the existence of parental influence, Cummins (1932) examined the age of the oldest son at marriage. He hypothesesd that the mothers had their first sons at relatively young age, and that this childhood memory of a young mother led the grown-up boys later to marry earlier with a younger woman. Samples from British *Who's Who* affirmed his hypothesis. Lidz (1960) suggested that the parental influence was actually effected through the childhood observation of complementary parental roles between the parents, or between the child and the parents. Since mother is usually the principal career of the child, the influence from the mother is expected to be more than from the father. Borchgrevink and Valvik's study (1983) supported that women chose partners to enter into same interactions that they had with their mothers.

Aron and colleagues (1974) surveyed 41 men and 31 women by attending the queue at the marriage license bureau. Respondents were asked of two questions on each of the six areas (openness, influence, dominance, responsiveness, trust, and playfulness) both about their part-ners and their fathers and mothers. The rating of one's partner was then compared with the rating of the parents. Both men and women subjects gave similar ratings to their partners as to their own mothers. This was viewed as a tendency for the subjects to repeat in their own marriage the kind of relationships they had with their mothers.

Jedlicka (1984) selected 3,500 brides and 3,000 grooms whose own parents differed in birthplace. Then the birthplaces of the parents were checked against the spouses'. Greater-than-expected frequencies were found between the birthplaces of the spouses, and that of the parents. Specifically, mothers appeared to have more influence on sons than on daughter, whereas the reverse was true for the fathers. In the same year, von der Lippe surveyed 76 married university students and professional social workers and again supported the claim of parental influence over the partner choice. She found that women choosing husbands like their fathers were more likely to report a good relationship with their mothers, and that one choosing a partner who resembled none or both of one's parents had greater capacity for emotional closeness.

Critique of Psychoanalytic Theory of Parental Influence

While no one would deny the positive or negative influence of their parents on the choice of partner, its weight and pathway remain obscure. Some placed emphasis on the parental roles during one's early childhood (Lidz, 1960), or the parental influence over the formation of the internalised and idealised self, whereas others suggested identification with parents (von der Lippe, 1965). The views on the importance of same-sex or opposite-sex parent for partner choice were not unitary either. The explanations varied, using non-specific parent-child interaction (Guntrip, 1961), specific parent-child relationship (von der Lippe, 1984; Jedlicka, 1984), mother-daughter relationship (Chasseguet-Smirgel, 1964; Chodorow, 1978; Borchgrevink & Valvik, 1983), or father-daughter relationship (Uddenberg et al, 1979).

Table 2.1 Psychological Models for Choice of Partner

Models	Theories	Authors
Psycho-dynamic	Electra & Oedipus Complex	Freud (1923); Commins (1932); Jung (1953); Gunstrip (1961); Chasseguet-Smirgel (1964); Aron et al. (1974); Chodorow (1978); von der Lippe (1984)
Personality Needs	Similarity	Burgess & Wallin (1953); Schellenberg (1960); Murstein (1961); Mehlman (1962); Banta & Hetherington (1963); Miller et al. (1966); Antill (1983); Lesnik-Oberstein & Cohen (1984)
	Complementarity	Winch (1955a, 1955b, 1958); Winch et al. (1955); Reik (1957); Rychlak (1965); Mathes & Moore (1983);
Sequential	Filter	Kerckhoff & Davis (1962)
	Wheel	Reiss (1960, 1988); Rubin (1976); Murstein (1970, 1976, 1987)
	Premarital Dyadic Formation	Lewis (1972, 1973)
Process	Interpersonal Process	Bolton (1961); Duck & Sants (1983); Femlee et al. (1990)
	Pathway	Cate et al. (1986); Cate (1992); Surra (1985, 1987)

The psychoanalytic investigations are apparently not systematic and vigorous enough. Selection of cases from British *Who's Who* (Commins, 1932) or from educated and professionals (von der Lippe, 1984) will have to answer seriously the question of validity. Another problem is about the dimension and construct being measured. Firstly, most these studies surveyed only one or both parties of the couple. Their views of the parents and partner were compared to their own views and to their views of the partner. It is the perceived similarity of the respondent that is being examined rather than an objective comparison. Secondly, most of the studies are with people who are going to marry or people who are newly wed. It will not be appropriate to extend any suggestion to those who failed or survived the marriage. Finally, the operational definitions of the construct of parental influence are problematic. Age at marriage of the oldest son is not good enough. They married at a younger age does not necessarily imply that they wanted a younger wife, by the influence of their mothers. Oldest sons are likely to be called on to work and support the family. They are less likely to remain longer in education than the younger brothers and therefore are less likely to marry at an older age. Since they married when they were young, they were likely to marry also a young wife. The use of birthplaces to ascertain the parental influence is another example of weak operational definitions. To infer from the matching of birthplaces is insignificant if not irrelevant. Even if differential parental influence on different-sex children in the aspect of birthplace has been established, it reduces the construct of parental influence to such a limited scope that it can hardly describe the generalised and often unconscious search for a partner who is like one or both parents.

The approach in essence is intra-psyche, and childhood-determinstic. It has very little space for situational factors of how one meets and chooses a partner. The child's own temperament, social skills and the development of other social relationships, and one's immediate socio-economic environment are all given no due considerations, but they are factors that could have shaped one's ideal self or ideal partner.

Theory of Personality Needs: Similarity Versus Complementarity

Complementarity In spite of different focuses among complementarity theorists, complementarity was said to exist when one partner has a high need and the other has a low need in the same personality area, and when one partner's need can be satisfied by the other partner, or when one partner can avoid behaviour that conflicts with the other partner. Winch and colleagues (1955) introduced two concepts of complementarity: the differences in intensity of identical needs (Type 1), and differences in kind of needs (Type 2); and three factor dimensions of complementarity: nurturance-receptivity, dominance-submissiveness, and achievement-vicariousness. Winch extended his theory that the congruence between personality needs and role specifications plays an important part in mate selection. In brief, Winch saw the gratification of needs as the focus of the intimate relationship, and these needs are a function of those unmet needs outside one's marriage. In a slightly different version, Reik (1957) theorised that one falls in love with someone who is different from oneself and who promises benefits that he or she cannot attain alone or with someone similar. He emphasised the exchange nature of the intimate relationship, which, according to Reik, is more linked with the sex roles than with the unmet needs outside marriage.

Similarity The theory holds that people select marital partners on the basis of whether they are similar to each other. Both daters and married couples were found to be similar in attitudes and values (Burgess & Wallin, 1953; Schellenberg, 1960), and personality (Antill, 1983). These similarities may reinforce the sense of togetherness and are more likely to reward each other in the course of interaction (Huston & Levinger, 1978).

More recent studies have not drawn firm conclusions, but have reconciled the disputes in some respects and added new knowledge to the situation under which the two hypotheses operate. Mathes and Moore (1983) have examined and supported Reik's (1957) complementarity theory of romantic love that one falls in love when one is dissatisfied with oneself and meets some of the opposite sex who has those characteristics that he or she desires but has been unable to achieve. An interpersonal checklist (Leary, 1957) and a self-esteem scale (Rosenberg, 1965) are used respectively for ideal and actual self assessment, and for distinguishing the high- and low-self-esteem groups. Overall, subjects were more attracted to peers embodying their own ideal characteristics than to those who did not. However, low-self-esteem subjects were found more likely to be attracted to romantic partners on the basis of Reikian complementarity while the high-self-esteem subjects were more likely to be attracted to romantic partners on the basis of actual similarity. In the Netherlands, Lesnik-Oberstein and Cohen (1984) analysed 177 volunteer couples on several psychological dimensions with the use of a number of tests. They suggest that similarity of cognitive style (reflection-impulsivity) and sensation seeking (experience seeking, disinhibition, and boredom susceptibility) may play a role in mate selection and in determining marital quality.

Critique of Theory of Personality Needs

The question whether "likes attract" or "opposites attract" is apparently over-simplified, and dichotomised, though very appealing to folk wisdom. First, it is not possible in the present stage of knowledge to identify all personality needs and whether they are similar or complementary between the couples. Individuals tend to interact with others living, working, and learning close to them, and hence are more likely to be limited in their opportunity to interact with people who are dissimilar to them. Similarity of personality need may, therefore, plays a less direct role in the actual decision-making of choosing a partner. While there is no proof that similarity of personality is a result of prolonged interaction, there is some evidence that similarity in values and world view can be affected through living together (Stephen, 1985), and that similarity alone does not distinguish couples who break up and who stay together (Hill et al, 1976).

On the other hand, although the complementarity theme is more developed and sophisticated than the similarity theme in allowing a consideration of exchange, and the involvement of the normative roles of the two sexes in that exchange process, there is no clear theoretical rationale to justify the inclusion of certain needs and the exclusion of others. Most complementarity studies (except Kerchhoff and Davis) use a normative approach, assuming the existence of certain needs and that these needs are complementary in nature among different couples. It is, however, very possible that what has been regarded as complementary by one group may not be regarded as complementary by another group. Finally, the two themes were originally attempts to explain how people fall in romantic love, and therefore may be necessary but not sufficient to explain the choice of a more permanent relationship. Even though some complementary elements are found in couples, it does not imply that they select each other for that reason, or on these grounds. In brief, the conceptualisation is questionable, and other researchers have failed to reproduce similar findings (Tharp, 1963; Murstein, 1976; Seyfried, 1977).

Sequential Theories

In response to the lack of theoretical clarity of the one dimensional analysis such as similarity and complementarity of personality needs, more complicated perspectives have been developed with increasing recognition that the process of mate selection cannot be reduced to a static single event, and that marriage is in fact preceded by different stages of courtship. In these different stages, there are different psychological variables of different level of importance, exerting influence over the stability of the relationship.

Filter Theory Kercekhoff and Davis (1962) studied dating pairs in college at the start and end of an 8-month period. The predictors vary according to the length of courtship. They have found that consensus and need complementarity are both important variables for the development of a relationhip. Value consensus seemed to have exerted greater influence in the early stage while later need complementarity becomes increasingly an important determinant of a stable and intimate relationship. This was indicated by value consensus as a predictor for those having dated for less than 18 months, and by need complementarity as a predictor for those having dated for 18 months or more. Similarity of social background variables, on the other hand, did not have a significant relationship with the progress of dating. This may suggest that subjects of both short and long-term dating groups have already selected partners of similar social backgrounds prior to the study. These findings have led to the suggestion of three groups of sequential "filters": the social characteristics, similarity in attitude and values, and need complementarity. Individuals filter or narrow down their prospective mates along the different stages with these factors.

Wheel Theory Reiss (1960, 1988) put forth a four-stage model of intimate relationship. There were thought to be four main stages for people to go through: rapport, self-revelation, mutual dependency, and intimacy need fulfillment. In the first stage, potential partners feel at ease and try to understand and communicate with one another. Supposedly, rapport can be developed out of a partner's perceived similarity of attitude and backgrounds. When rapport is established, individuals begin to reveal themselves (e.g. values, political and religious belief, personal details and experience) more freely. Social variables like social class may influence in this stage the extent and style of self-disclosure (Rubin, 1976). What follows self-revelation is a relationship that is characterised by mutual dependency. In this stage, particular partners take on significance for each other because certain rewards are only obtainable from a particular one, and not from others. Those who successfully pass through these stages will come to a stage where the relationship is evaluated according to whether it can meet intimacy needs. Factors like culture and one's social role may influence the way these needs are expressed and met.

Stimulus-Value-Role Model Murstein (1970, 1976, 1987) elaborated on the sequential model and has proposed a Stimulus-Value-Role (SVR) theory. He believed that couples are attracted to each other because of the equality of exchange of assets and liabilities [physical, social, and economic] that each one possesses. The path to marriage or living together has to undergo three main stages. The first stage is stimulus (S), in which potential partners are constantly evaluating the other's physical and socio-economic attributes. Satisfaction at this stage is not based on absolute equality of each and every characteristic, but rather an approximate equality of the total. When approximate equality is achieved, they move to the second stage. In this stage, personal basic values that they have (e.g. social and political) are revealed during the increased interaction, and compatibility is sought before they can exchange more intimate details. Relationship is not likely to be maintained only on the basis of value consensus. Eventually, one must take into account how each partner perceives the function of the other lover, companion, housekeeper, parents.

His early model stressed the influence of different variables in different stages, but later Murstein reformulated his model so that relationship variables are stage-specific (1987). Some variables are more influential in affecting courtship. Stimulus variables are more important in the first stage, while value-related variables have more influence in the second stage, and role-related variables are the most influential in the final stage. According to Murstein, couples who have successfully navigated these three stages are more likely to have a mutually satisfying intimate relationship and to remain in marriage, than those who have not.

Premarital Dyadic Formation Framework (PDF) Lewis (1972, 1973) proposed six sequences for the development of intimate heterosexual relationships. The six sequential processes are perceiving similarities, achieving pair rapport, inducing self-disclosure, role taking, achieving interpersonal role-fit, and achieving "dyadic crystallisation". The first three processes are similar in nature to the stages proposed by other sequential theorists, but the fourth processes is distinct in that role-fit can be achieved through either personality similarity, role complementarity or need complementary, and the pattern differs between couples. The final stage is characterised by progressive involvement, dyadic functioning, boundary establishment, pair commitment, and couple identity formation. It is in this phase that couples are becoming increasingly inter-dependent in more permanent relationships.

Critique of Sequential Theories

The early form of sequential theory was relatively simplistic. There was no clarification of the exact stages of development, nor mention of what other factors, apart from value consensus and need complementarity, could have been an important influence. The inter-relationship between these variables is unclear and it is not known whether it is the changing psychological needs, the effect of other variables, or the combination of both that leads to the increasing or diminishing influence of a particular variable.

While it might be true for some couples to have progressed through a journey of intimacy before making a marriage commitment, it appears that the classification of the stages is arbitrary and without proper conceptual or theoretical justification (Rubin & Levinger, 1974). The presumption that situations leading to the marriage decision must provide increasing intimacy has been challenged by the evidence that some relationship lack the sense of intimacy right from the beginning of the marital relationship (Cuber & Harroff, 1966), and that working-class couples may quickly move to marriage by non-intimate events like a difficult home environment or unwanted pregnancy (Rubin, 1976). The implicit assumption that need complementarity or compatibility is the driving force for marriage has received only limited empirical support, but has ignored to a large extent the interaction between partners and other situational factors (Huston et al, 1981).

Among the critics, Stephen (Stephen & Markman, 1983; Stephen, 1984, 1985) is most outstanding in opposing the mechanical development of the dyadic relationship along a S-V-R line. He argued that values were not independent and separate from personality traits, and has found no significant difference in the correlation of expressed values between different couple groups. Murstein (1987) has reinterpreted this point as supporting rather than conflicting evidence by arguing that most of the subjects in Stephen's studies were past the V Stage and in the R stage, and therefore will not be significant different across different couple groups, but will be as a whole significantly higher than the stranger group.

This has raised an even more serious problem - the operational definition of stages, which is more obvious in S-V-R than in other sequential theories. Murstein has classified the first contact as S stage, 2-7 contacts as V stage, and 8 and more contacts as R stage. Such a definition is arbitrary and would have placed most subjects of the dyadic research indiscriminately in R stage. This theoretic consideration has given researchers little opportunity to research and validate the first two stages, while the third stage actually encompasses most of the subjects. Classifying stages in this way is convenient, but has not dealt with the serious risk from systematic bias which arises of the arbitrary division based on only very a small number of contacts. Other sequential theorists (e.g. Leigh et al, 1987) have expressed difficulty in determining the stages. In many cases, the subjects' views of their own stages of development has not been taken into account.

Levinger, Senn and Jorgensen (1970) did not find any linear or curvilinear association between value consensus and courtship progress, nor a strong relationship between need complementarity and courtship progress. Rubin and Levinger (1974) rightly pointed out that in the accounts of the progress of an intimate relationship, sequential theory lacks the specificity of the exact filtering process. In spite of all these difficulties, sequential theory brings a major contribution to the study of dyadic relationship in that it is a process model, emphasising the involvement of different psychosocial variables (e.g. attractiveness, value consensus, personality needs) which exert their influence differentially during different stages of development. Further empirical validation is need to clarify and improve the definition the stages used, and to explore what major psychosocial variables are involved and what the exact inter-relationships are.

Interpersonal Process Model

This model also attempts to address the issue of differential influence of different factors, but is different from sequential theories in two major ways. Firstly, although similarity of social variables and attitude, and other static factors play a role in the course of the relationship, it is actually the interaction between the partners themselves that shapes the development to an intimate relationship (Duck & Sants, 1983). The interaction is tied to, but not predetermined by personal attributes, together with the social and physical environment that the partners are in (Kelley et al, 1983). Secondly, the model allows multiple causes at different levels, and thus multiple pathways instead of a relatively straight sequence in the progression to a marriage or intimate relationship.

Bolton's (1961) work has been regarded as one of the early works that support the idea of multiple pathways to marriage. He identified five main types of development that characterised the progression to marriage: personality meshing, expediency-centred, identity clarification, relation-centred, and pressure and intrapersonal. Each type has its own characteristics and is influenced by different factors. For instance, the expediency-centred type exerts a strong pressure to marry by one or both partners, and the pressure is related to personality problems or identity crisis. In contrast, the relationship-centred type is characterised by initial superficial commitment which is gradually adjusted and built to deeper commitment over "high" and "low" in the relationship.

Cate et al. (1986) further developed the idea of pathway and process, and discerned three main types of pathways to marriage among 50 newly-wed couples. Prolonged courtship is a slow, up-and-down progression to marriage, correlated with conflict at all premarital stages, and ambivalence during serious dating. These conflicts and ambivalences may be related to parental opposition. Accelerated courtship takes place when there is less conflict, and more compatible interaction is catalysed by external factors like older age, and the perception of parental approval. Intermediate courtship is the one "between" the other two paths. It is characterised by low level of conflict, initial hesitancy, and slow movement to commitment. The initial hesitancy may signify other alternative relationships which have to be disengaged in order to proceed with this new relationship.

Surra (1985, 1987) in a similar fashion replicated Cate's three pathways, but found a fourth path, accelerated-arrest, which was similar to the accelerated courtship but had a downturn in commitment at a later stage in the relationship before marriage. Surra also found that the activity levels between the couples, and between the partner and his / her own social network varied for different types of pathway. Although as a whole, partners were becoming more engaged with each other and less engaged with their social network, the disengagement was more rapid for the accelerated-arrested couples than for the accelerated (only) ones. Pairs in prolonged courtship maintained their level of activity with their network, while the intermediate type had more network contact and less companionship with the partner.

On the other hand, Femlee et al. (1990) studied the dissolution of relationships and found that some dyadic factors like love, ambivalence, sexual intimacy, time spent together, and maintenance behaviour predicted the break-up. Only dyadic variables and social network variables, but not individual variables were related to the stability of the relationship.

Critique of Interpersonal Process Model

The interpersonal process framework can be seen as an integrated attempt to incorporate individual variables (psychological traits and attributes), dyadic variables (interaction and communication), social network (other social relationship), and circumstantial variables into the analysis of the development of intimate relationship. The framework is more versatile and advanced than the early assumptions of unconscious driving forces for a partner similar to one's parent, or the active conscious search for a compatible partner. The interpersonal process that this framework portrays is certainly more complicated, but flexible than the sequential theory. It appears to be more promising than other psychological perspectives for our understanding of the development of the intimate relationship and the mate choice. However, one major problem is that it has just not gone far enough in considering the socio-economic and genetic aspects of mate choice. Psychological process or interaction is the focus of a "snapshot" without due considerations being given to the socio-economic situations under which the psychological process is taking place.

Conclusion

The process models are more dynamic than the classical theories of childhood complexes, and personal needs, but their verification may demand more resources in the long term follow-up of a representative sample. The concept of different stages of an intimate relationship is perhaps the least developed and there has been no further suggestion about the mode of progress, be it sequential, overlapping, or differential pathways.

It will be fair to note that the process models are still being developed and there is no process model that may be adopted, with confidence, for psychiatric patients. It will be probably too ambitious to apply it while the contention and argument continues in the respect of normal population. The psycho-social context under which acquaintance and intimacy developed is largely unknown for the patients. Before we can come to the stage of model building, we must first try to find the answers for some very basic questions: is it the same kind of attraction and romantic love that the patient and their spouses experienced as ordinary pairs; what were their social situations before they came to know each other marriage; where did they first meet; were they similar in terms of family background, opinions and values, and social habits before they married; what were their considerations and reasons for marriage.

Sociological Investigations of Mate Selection

Samples of married couples, or more exactly those married couples who remained in the marriage, are found to be similar across a wide range of social variables such as race, religion, value, attitude, education, and social class (Epstein & Guttman, 1984). These similarities suggest the crucial part played by social factors in shaping the mate selection pattern.

Propinquity

Early sociological attempts centred around residential propinquity (Katz & Hill, 1958; Kerckhoff, 1956). People of similar socio-economic background tend to segregate themselves from others who are different from them. In this way, the social environment (school, neighbourhood, workplace etc.) from which a mate is chosen tend to be homogeneous. Potential mates of similar social background, aptitude, and activity level are provided with a greater-than-chance opportunity to relate to each other. Geographical propinquity may be just a reflection of a larger systematic social stratification.

Exchange Theory

Exchange theorists (Blau, 1964; Edwards, 1969) considered human subjects to be in constant exchange of their resources. Resources can be of two types: cultural resources and socio-economic resources. Cultural resources include values and norms (personal, familial, or cultural), life-style, leisure activities, interest, life experience. Although personal evaluation of resources may vary from a person to another, there is a normative view on socio-economic resources which include not only the monetary asset, but also the indivisible value that can be "purchased" through the market, like beauty, pleasure, security, and health. People with similar cultural resources, knowingly or unknowingly, tend to have a more mutually rewarding relationship than otherwise. Not only are they more likely to confirm each other's behaviour and attitude, but also that they share a common schema of discourse which promotes mutual understanding (DiMaggio & Mohr, 1985).

Becker (1981) has argued that the exchange of paid and domestic labour within the family would be most rewarding, and hence suggested a negative assortative mating on economic status. Although the strict division of paid and domestic work has been less obvious during this century due to the increasing involvement of women in economic activities, it still holds true that men are in control of much of the economic resources of a family, and are structurally in a more advantaged position. They can aim for economic compatibility, or domestic and sexual services that they value (Schoen & Wooldredge, 1989).

Among members of either sex, those who possess greater economic resources may be more able to choose from available pool of partners, and are less willing to marry those with comparatively undesirable or non-normative characteristics. People tend to marry others from a similar social background partly because they may be rejected by those who have greater resources than they have, and they are more likely to reject those with fewer resources.

Critique of Exchange Theory

The exchange perspective rests on the idea of equity and a reciprocal relationship between the sexes. In the first place, the equity notion is based on differential control of valued resources (Wolfe, 1959; Blood & Wolfe,

1960). In the latter, the reciprocity of roles and resources is regarded as functional for the stability of the relationship (Parsons, 1956). This notion resembles ideas of individual complementarity and fails to recognise the very different nature of economic and non-economic resources, and the unequal power relationship within and outside marriage. The assumption of equity, as shall be seen, is unnecessary and has little empirical support. In the second place, non-economic resources are not characterised by self-regeneration and accumulation, and are not standard units and means for exchange as are economic resources. In brief, they are not "convertible" in the same way. Domestic work which is so often regarded as one of the non-economic but valued commodities is often routine, boring, manual, non-creative, isolating, and unpaid. The material and non-material rewards derived from domestic labour is incomparable with those from a paid job.

Although there have been reports of more flexible attitudes and a gradual increase in husbands' involvement in domestic tasks in Britain (Gershuny & Jones, 1987), working women continue to carry the burden of domestic tasks (Oakley, 1974; Pahl, 1971, 1984; Martin & Roberts, 1984). Gershuny (1982) reported that the unpaid work of employed wives does not decline in proportion to their increase in paid work, and the British Social Attitudes Survey (Jowell & Witherspoon, 1985) did not find an egalitarian division of domestic work between couples who both work. On the other hand, Laite and Halfpenny's study in Macclesfield and Blackburn (1987) found that women were most burdened when they had to look after young children and to be in part-time employment. The unequal situation in domestic responsibility did not seem to alter when women are in full-time employment (Pleck, 1985) or when men are unemployed (Morris, 1985). This evidence suggests that the exchange relationship is not one of equality, and that women are disadvantaged. Feminist writers argue that the oppression and disadvantaged position of the women in western society stems from a patriarchal system of values and roles which seek to maintain men's supremacy (Mainardi, 1970; Barret, 1980; Hartman, 1981).

Marriage Market

The second approach deals more with the availability of mating pools, and the circumstances people bring to the marriage market and result in subsequent mating patterns. Individuals are in an advantaged position if they can have sufficient mate choice, and they will have little motivation to expand their available pools of potential mates by including people whom they consider to have dissimilar or undesirable traits. On the other hand, people with non-normative trait or less desired characteristics are more likely to expand their limited pool and to show a greater willingness to marry persons with dissimilar personal and social characteristics, or to remain unmarried. Most partnerships that take place in the "market" are formed on the ground of equity. Individuals tend to avoid inequity and to achieve equity by choosing similar partners (Walster et al, 1966; Murstein, 1976), but there are always some people who could not make such a match and remain single for different reasons. When compared by sex and race, black women are found to be the most disadvantaged (Spanier & Glick, 1980; Guttentag & Secord, 1983; Wilson, 1987; Tucker & Taylor, 1989).

There are different definitions of the marriage market. It can be the geographical composition of the marriageable population (an predetermined age range) as a whole (Goldman et al, 1984), or marriageable population of local areas and districts (Ramsoy, 1966; Peach, 1974), or even educational institutions (Scott, 1965; Reiss, 1965; Bayer, 1972). Analysis based on national demographic data is prone to bias due to possible regional differences, and the fact that even in the same area, access to the marriage market and the availability of potential mates may vary from person to person. Residential proximity has one time been regarded as important in mate selection (Eckland, 1968), while educational institutions have been receiving more and more attention.

Educational reforms might have given rise to the importance of educational institutions in the marriage market. Most young people of similar age, but different sex can come to school on a daily basis. Girls have more equal access to education than they did before. As a result, schools and colleges have become one of the major pools where the sex ratio has the least effect. Classroom and outside-classroom activities provide excellent opportunities for the testing out, and reinforcement of matching on attitudes, interest, and personal and cultural resources. Exposure to common educational experience and life experience in this developmental stage will also help form the social circle which consists of relatively homogeneous groups in terms of the students' characteristics. Becoming used to a particular kind of interaction pattern may increase the likelihood of later choosing a partner with a similar educational background, or even one from their former course-mates.

This holds particularly true when the more educated remain in their education as they get older, and hence are less available in the marriage market for those who have less education and who have joined the workforce in an earlier age. In contrast, when the more educated become available mates, those who join the pools earlier might already have selected a partner.

Kalmijn (1991) has used log-linear models to avoid the probable bias of marginal distribution of status homogamy between couples, and has argued that, in the United States, education (which is defined as an achieved status) is a more important boundary in marriage selection than social-class origins and that genuine educational homogamy between couples has increased over time. It is unclear whether this thesis may equally well be applied to Britain. The economic recession might have forced more people of marriageable age to live with their own parents, and more people out of work, hence producing a less mobile population. The impact of a static housing market may also make a contribution. Consequently, residential propinquity and social origin may currently have a bigger effect on the timing and selection of a partner.

Critique of Marriage Market

There has been no real "marriage market" in economy because the boundary of available pool of potential mates varies according to different regions, districts and cultural groups. Mortensen (1988) put forth numeric models for voluntary matching in marriage and employment market and he admitted that there could be uncertainties in the structure of the market:

> ...unstable structures can form when matching requires time, is costly, and takes place under conditions of uncertainty both because it is not rational to wait indefinitely for the perfect partner and because experience is required to discover the value of a specific partnership... Unfortunately, in the case of marriage, no indicator of match quality seems to exist that would permit one to obtain an answer using the techniques applied in the case of worker-employer relationships. At this point in time, one can only speculate. (p.S238-39)

The information about the market is incomplete and the choice of mate is not necessarily the result of constant evaluation of self and potential partner's relative position in the pool. The choice may not always be a rational one. Yet it seems that education itself has become an important factor that relaxes or restricts the boundary of potential mates and influences the timing of becoming available in the pool. The effect of education on mate choice seems to be clearer in the people who spent more time in educational institutions, and less clearer in those who received less education.

Both the exchange and market approach stress the bartering of valuable resources between partners, which treats an intimate relationship basically from consumer's view. Although this perspective does not exclude other non-sociological influences, psychological and interactional variables are partly ordered by a predetermined set of sociological variables. This consumptive view is not consistent with the developmental view that the additive nature of interactions between the partners is so essential to the formation and stability of an intimate relationship, or the evolutionist view in which exchange process is seen as reproductive rather than consumptive in nature.

Conclusion

Choice of partner is constrained by the socio-economic situation that one is in. People are more likely to choose partners who are similar in socio-economic background. In a sense, one's tangible resources expand or restrict one's available pool of potential mates. If that is the case for normal population, by investigating the extent of such social homogamy among patients who suffer from more severe forms of mental illness, we shall be able to see how far the illness itself and its debilitating consequence alter such a pattern. The initial hypothesis is that people with severe form of illness like schizophrenia have their social exposure reduced because of reduced motivation to relate to people and deficits in interpersonal skills, which in turn produces a smaller pool of potential mates.

3 Genetics and Evolution

Genetics and Psychiatric Illness

The twentieth century has witnessed growing interest in the study of genetic variation and heredity. With discoveries and advancement in genetic technology, the Mendelian laws of Gregor Mendel have received revived attention. The first law, the law of segregation, states that there are two discrete heredity elements for a single character, offspring receiving one of the two elements from each parent. Mendel's second law, known as the law of independent assortment, states that when there is inheritance of two traits, each with two elements, the elements for each trait assort independently of the elements for the other trait.

Molecular biology bestowed new meaning upon heredity by discovering that a gene is the coded stretch of deoxyribonucleic acid (DNA) located in chromosomes in the nucleus of a cell. Chromosomes are in pairs, one deriving from each parent. Alternative forms of genes (alleles) are at the same locus on the matching chromosomes. It is the gene(s) at a different location (loci) that determine(s) the manifestation and heredity of certain biological characteristics. Huntington's disease followed the simple Mendelian principle of transmission in the way that a single dominant defective gene from either parent is sufficient to bring about the disease. The pattern of transmission can be spotted from the family history long before a molecular biological technique was able to locate the specific gene on chromosome 4. Another disease, Phenylketonuria (PKU) is transmitted through a recessive mode in which manifestation only takes place in the offspring of two carriers. However, many physical diseases like Alzheimer's disease, epilepsy, coronary heart disease, and most of the psychoses are very likely to be polygenic and do not abide by the Mendelian principles.

Since DNA can replicate itself in exactly the same biologically coded structure, genetic variability is possible only under four main circumstances, namely: mutation, natural selection, migration, and inbreeding and non-random mating. The first two conditions take perhaps millions of years for the nature to alter and transmit a genotype while migration depends very much on the variability of genotypes between the two populations that one comes from and to. With relative ease of transport and fluidity of the population, it is also difficult to demarcate the effect of migration. Inbreeding normally takes many generations to demonstrate the effects of homogeneity of genotypes. Human species cannot be mani-pulated like laboratory animals, where there can be continuous and systematic back or cross mating within selected families.

The role of heredity and genetics is particularly relevant to the etiology and epidemiology of psychiatric disorder, and the knowledge of genetics has considerable implications for the understanding, treatment, and prevention of pathology. The history of genetic studies can be divided into old and new eras with the development of DNA recombinant technology as the watershed in the 1980s. The old era was characterised by the classical approach of twins, family, and adoption studies, and has received, in general, support from more recent studies with more advanced genetic technology. The new era is being marked by more advanced techniques of molecular genetics like Restriction Fragment Length Polymorphism (RFLP), Polymerase Chain Reaction and gene deliveries. It will be shown later that this century and the next one are going to be revolutionised by the genetic discoveries, which are bringing about excitement as well as ethical dilemma.

Classical Approach

Twin Study Monozygotic twins (MZ) generally exhibited much higher concordance rates for schizophrenia than Dizygotic twins (DZ) – approximately between four to six folds - in different studies (Table 3.1).

Twin studies before the 1970s in general yielded higher MZ and DZ rates than later studies. This can be explained partly by the over-correction for age, inclusion of a wider or narrower definition of schizophrenia, the difference in the sex of the twin pairs, different sources of samples (ward, local register or national register), and different severity and chronicity of the samples. Earlier methods have been criticised for higher risk of systematic bias due to non-blindfold design, lack of adequate control groups, and the lack of diagnostic precision. When improvements were made with regard to these areas, a lower MZ and DZ rate was evident.

Although from these figures one can see that genetics is beyond doubt a significant factor, MZ twins did not have 100% nor did DZ twins have 50% concordance as Mendelian principles would have suggested. MZ twins differ from DZ twins not only in genetic structure, but also in prenatal and peri-natal environment. In the case of DZ fetus, nutritional supply is separate and the embryo's environment can be very different. Same or similar post-natal circumstances cannot be assumed for MZ and DZ twins either. MZ twins, because of biological resemblance in early years (height, weight, appearance, voice) are more likely than DZ twins to receive similar treatment from their social environment.

Table 3.1 Concordance of Twins

Schizophrenia :	**MZ (%)**	**DZ (%)**
Luxenburger (1928)	58	-
Rosanoff et al (1934) [a]	61	13
Essen-Moller (1941) [a]	64	15
Kallmann (1946) [b]	86	15
Slater (1953) [a]	65	14
Kringlen (1967)[d]	28 / 38	6 / 14
Fischer (1971)	64	27
Tienari (1975) [b]	36	14
Gottesman & Shields (1972)	58	12
Gottesman & Shields (1982)	46	14
Kendler & Robinette (1983) [cd]	31	6
Bipolar Affective Disorder :		
Bertelsen et al (1977)	79	19

[a] same-sex twins
[b] male twins only
[c] corrected for age
[d] schizophrenia spectrum disorder

Adoption Studies Adoption studies also support a genetic contribution to the etiology of schizophrenia. Heston (1966) managed to interview forty-seven adoptees at the average age of thirty-six and then compared them to fifty normal controls matched for sex, type of placement and care. These forty-seven adoptees, during their first two weeks of life, were placed away from their mothers who were schizophrenic and were hospitalised during their pregnancy. Five out of forty seven were diagnosed as schizophrenic cases, arriving at a 16.6% morbidity rate after correction for age. Nine cases were found to have sociopathic personality disorder, and thirteen to have other psychiatric disorders. In another study, the biological relatives of the thirty three schizophrenic adoptees were found to be four and a half times as likely as the biological relatives of the control group to be also schizophrenic (Kety et al, 1968). Rosenthal and Kety (1968) traced the Danish national register of all adoptions between 1924 and 1947, and had judged sixty-nine adoptees at least one of whose parent was psychotic (56 schizophrenic, 13 affective disorder). Of these adoptees, three were assessed as schizophrenics, six with borderline schizophrenia, three with schizoid personality, and one with paranoid personality.

One major limitation of adoption studies is that these adoptee groups are usually children of in-patient mothers or parents whose clinical conditions are considered as severe and chronic. There has been no available information of those biological parents with less severe forms of illness. Besides, parents who give up their children for adoption are more likely to be referred by social services professionals for psychiatric screening than parents who retain their children. Therefore even the control group will have higher morbidity risk than the general population. This probably explains why when Lowing and others (1983) re-analyzed the Danish samples with DSM-III criteria, the control group showed 10% cases as having spectrum disorder; a figure that may suggest the adoptee group in general is different from the normal population. It would be much better methodologically to study adopted twins reared apart as in normal population (Bouchard & McGue, 1990), but it is simply not possible in the case of treated population..

Family Studies Higher morbidity risk has been found among family members of the patient group than in the control group in respect of anxiety and panic disorder (Crowe et al, 1983; Noyes et al, 1987), bipolar disorder (Weissman et al, 1984), alcoholism (Pitts & Winokur, 1966), and schizophrenia (Gottesman & Bertelsen, 1989a; 1989b). One major prospective study was done by Mednick and Schulsinger (1968) who followed up 207 children born of a schizophrenic mother in the period 1941-1954, and compared this group to a control group of 104 subjects. By 1967, no schizophrenia was found either in the proband or the control. By 1980 (Parnas et al, 1982), thirteen had schizophrenia, and five had committed suicide in the proband group but there was only one control subject who had schizophrenia and none committed suicide.

Gottesman (1991) pooled the figures of 40 studies between 1920 and 1987 in Western Europe and compiled the lifetime risk of developing schizophrenia among different family members. MZ twins and the offspring of dual mating (two patient parents) were highest, respectively 48% and 46%. First degree relatives were in the range 6% (parents) to 17% (DZ twins, and siblings with one schizophrenic parent); second degree relatives ranged from 2% (uncle/aunt) to 6% (half siblings). Other relationships like first cousins and spouses of patients are considered to be at only twice the risk of the general population. The genetic factor is clearly evident from the outstanding risk of MZ twins and offspring of dual mating, while DZ twins have a much lower rate. The familial link is also evident in the fact that first-degree relatives have a higher risk than second-degree relatives. The positive relationship between closeness of kinship and increasing risk seems to hold when the relationships are broadly categorised into first and second-degree relatives. However, a uniform or similar rate has not been reached for all sub-groups under the same category. Considerable within-group variation is found between children (13%) and parents (6%), although they are actually the two ends of a genetic relationship. Clearly, as far as schizophrenia is concerned, children are subject to other factors like parenting while the parents are less likely to be aversely affected by the children. DZ twins (17%) have almost twice the risk of siblings (9%), although the genetic linkage should be the same for both of them. This may suggest non-genetic elements at work within the family, but there is little agreement about the nature and importance of these non-genetic factors.

It is noteworthy that not all studies have comparable diagnostic criteria. There are worries that some earlier studies might have adopted diagnostic criteria, which are judged by modern standards to be less strict. Pope et al. (1983) with the use of DSM-III criteria did not find any morbidity in one hundred and ninety nine first-degree relatives of schizophrenics. Another study (Abrams & Taylor, 1983) found only 1.6% lifetime prevalence with a sample of the 128 first degree relatives of schizophrenia sufferers. McGuffin (1988) argued that the low estimate did not rule out the role of genetics of the disorder since the figure of probands should always be compared to the control subjects, who, according to more restrictive criteria, can be as low as 0.2% (Kendler et al, 1985). Therefore a lower estimate is not sufficient to invalidate the older studies, but it certainly makes comparison and meta-analysis difficult. In some situations, the use of different but valid diagnostic criteria can result in different classifications (McGuffin et al, 1982).

There are three probable explanations about the non-genetic components of mental illness, namely psychosocial factors, viral and organic hypotheses, and heterogeneity of disease type. Psychosocial factors include those psychological and social conditions, particularly the stressors, which serve to trigger off or buffer against the predisposition. DZ twins have a higher risk than ordinary siblings developing disorders because DZ twins are more likely to be treated similarly than siblings who are already different in order and age. Psychosocial factors may also explain why MZ and the offspring of parents both of whom have schizophrenia do not have a near to hundred percent risk.

The viral and organic hypotheses draw support from the disproportionally high number of schizophrenic patients born in winter (Machon et al, 1983; Watson et al, 1984a), suggests that the disorder may be a direct latent result of season-related viral attack on the neurotransmitter system such as dopamine, norepinephrine, or serotonin. This hypothesis, however, succeeds in explaining why people living under the same roof have higher risk of developing the disorder, but fails to explain why professionals who are in constant contact with patient groups do not have higher morbidity risk. It is unreasonable to assume that mental health workers have a higher immunity or lower vulnerability to this viral attack. Partial support also comes from the study of lateral ventricular size of twins, relatives and patients themselves (Reveley et al, 1982, 1984; Schulsinger et al, 1984), which suggested that viral infection of a certain kind was responsible for changes in the lateral ventricular size of the discordant relatives of patients. Unfortunately, other studies of ventricular size did not support this argument (McGuffin et al, 1987; Farmer et al, 1987). Also, there has been speculation that birth trauma may be related to the development of schizophrenia (Pollin & Stabenau, 1968; McNeill & Kaij, 1978), but in Gottesman and Shields' review (1982), there was no convincing replication of these studies.

Certain studies (Gottesman & Bertelsen, 1989b) did not find any increased risk for mental illness among the offspring of parents at least one of whom suffered from reactive psychosis. Instead of arguing against the lack of genetic evidence, one may argue that there may be different types of disease of different etiologies but which are currently under the same diagnosis. After all, the similarity of symptoms or syndromes does not necessarily imply the same etiology. Current epidemiological studies are based on the conventional assumption of homogeneity of diagnostic type, and this assumption is subject to challenge. Crow (1980, 1985) postulated that there were actually two types of schizophrenia. Type I features positive symptoms, good response to neuroleptic treatment, and normal computed tomographic brain scan (CT) results. Type II disorder is associated with negative symptoms, poor response to neuroleptic treatment, and enlarged cerebral ventricular size. He suggested that Type I is caused by dopaminergic abnormality and that Type II disorder was caused by infection, is more severe, and genetically linked. On the other hand, Murray et al (1985) suggested that, of those who have been diagnosed as being schizophrenic, the illnesses of those without family history were in fact caused by mainly environmental factors, whereas some others were mainly genetically influenced. No confirmation of these suggestions of heterogeneity is possible at the present moment, and will have to await the results of further research.

Genetic Technologies Advanced molecular technology has transformed the study of genetics. Simple observation on phenotypic variation of plants, birds and insects has been abandoned and a wide range of studies and applications in insect, plant, animal, and human biology has been launched.

There are three main types of genetic probes. When an abnormal protein is found to be closely connected with an illness, investigations can then go into the gene that codes for the protein production in question. In this way, investigators have been able to locate the defective gene for Lesch-Nyhan syndrome, which is characterised by motor defects, speech difficulty, and self-mutilating behaviour (Gibbs & Caskey, 1987). Since not all gene metabolisms are readily understood, it is always difficult to ascertain the role of the protein and that of the other possible metabolic concomitants. Another alternative involves the use of a presumed "culprit" gene, or a distinct biological marker that is associated with the gene or "linked" with the product of a gene. When the region responsible for such a link is known, this will enable a more direct search for the defective gene in a particular region, thus greatly narrowing down the search. With the use of this method, the gene responsible for Alzheimer's disease was located near to the beta-amyloid gene which causes beta-amyloid protein accumulation in the brains of patients suffering from the disease (St George-Hyslop et al, 1987). The third type of probe uses fragments of genomic DNA cleaved by restriction enzymes. The genomic DNAs of different necleotide base sequences are cleaved into fragments of different length, and then mapping techniques like electrophoresis (Harris, 1969; Snell & Wilkins, 1986; Bustamante et al, 1993; Maule, 1998) and Southern Blot (Southern, 1975) are used to determine the differences between two genomes. The cleaving process is often referred to as Restriction Fragment Length Polymorphism (RFLP) (Botstein et al, 1980) and has been widely applied in DNA fingerprinting in forensic science. Molecular genetics makes it possible to have linkage or association analysis and eventually localise the defective gene, and thus the group at risk (Yates & Conner, 1986; Lander & Schork, 1994; Lander & Kruglyak, 1995). Hopefully, by comparing those who do not develop with those who have developed the disorder within the affected gene group, we may understand better the possible situations (including environmental influence) under which the disorder developed or was inhibited.

The use of DNA markers in genetic linkage studies has brought about new understanding to the cause of certain physical illness including polycystic kidney disease (Reeder et al, 1985), cystic fibrosis (White et al, 1985), and muscular dystrophy (Davies et al, 1983). In psychiatry, the state of knowledge is still developing, and the degree of genetic influence on various disorders is not always firmly established yet. For example, genetic influence is more certain in Huntington's disease (Gusella et al, 1983) and Alzheimer's disease (Goate et al, 1991; Sherrington et al, 1995; Rogaev et al, 1995; Wragg et al, 1996; Carr et al, 1997), than in schizophrenia (Sherrington et al, 1988), and bipolar affective disorder. The Amish study in Pennsylvania (Egeland et al, 1987) has been able to localise a gene at the tip of the short arm of chromosome 11 that is closely linked to manic-depressive disorder. The RFLP together with the use of segregation analyses of family pedigree has led to the suggestion of an autosomal dominant mode of transmission. In another study, Baron and colleagues (1987) found differently that the defective gene was possibly localised in the X-chromosome among a Israeli population.

Although recent studies appear to offer promises for decoding the secret of functional psychoses, existing different and often conflicting results have to be tolerated at least for some time. The involvement of which chromosome where the susceptibility genes are thought to be located remains contentious for bipolar disorder (Pekkarinen et al, 1995; Dawson et al, 1995; Blackwood et al, 1996; Freimer et al, 1996) and schizophrenia (Straub et al, 1995; Moises et al, 1995; Schwab et al, 1995; Pulver et al, 1995; Lin et al, 1995; SCLG, 1996). While the differences could be due to errors and differences in both the difference in sample and procedure, it is equally possible that there are different etiological disorders which are currently classified under the same diagnostic category.

The molecular genetic approach has clearly begun to demonstrate great potential for the understanding of the etiology of a wide range of diseases. It has at least three advantages over twins, adoption, family, and pedigree studies. The classical approach, in showing the existence of a possible genetic factor, did not provide further information as to where and what the genetic problems were, but the gene approach did. Second, not all the people with the defective gene develop the disorder. This could have resulted in the variation of the estimate of prevalence rates, and even an incorrect conclusion that heredity was not operating in a particular group. Gene approach contributes significantly to the identification of cases and potential cases who either have not yet developed into detectable illness or are just the carriers. Thirdly, gene approach offers a clear indication of the direction of prevention and treatment which classical studies lacked, although the effectiveness is more apparent in some diseases like Severe Combined Immunodeficiency Disease (SCID) than others. With techniques of genetic engineering, animals with a specific genetic defect and phenotype can be bred and tested for specific diagnostic probe and treatment before clinical trial on human beings.

No matter how promising the molecular approach appears to be, it is certainly not without problems and difficulties. The biochemical effects and pathways of most of the genes remain unknown. Even when a defective gene is localised, very little has been known as to when and how that gene has its effects. As in the study of bipolar affective disorder stated above, it is perfectly possible in the case of polygenic or multi-factorial mode of transmission, that more than one gene is responsible; or in a more complicated situation, different genes may be affected in different individuals but still lead to similar clinical manifestations. Pardes et al. (1989) called this "nonallelic genetic heterogeneity". On the other hand, theoretically, there can be cases without a genetic base, yet with similar clinical conditions, though technically one may never know whether a case is really without a genetic basis or is caused by another defective gene which has not yet been discovered.

Among geneticists the degree of optimism varies. While most researchers agree that environmental factors exercise at least a moderate influence on mental disorders, Crow (1984, 1986, 1988) argued for a purely genetic and biological base of the mental disorder. He ruled out the possibility of environmental influence on the ground that adoptees away from the family in which schizophrenia was present did not have a reduced risk, and that the onset of schizophrenia is unrelated to the onset of illness in siblings. He went on to argue that the near 50% concordance for schizophrenia of MZ twins was due to genetic rather than environmental factors. What he hypothesised was that schizophrenia is a genetic disorder relating to the arrested development of cerebral asymmetries (resulting in cognitive impairment), and that the psychosis gene has characteristics of a viral sequence expressed in episodes of the disorder. According to him, it is the gene that determines the timing, the episodes, and the overall illness behaviour.

Molecular studies added strength to the gene hypothesis with further refinement, but still there was no conclusive result. For example, in the genome studies of schizophrenia, there were suggestions of chromosome 22 (Pulver et al, 1994; Coon et al, 1994), chromosome 4 (Barr et al, 1994), chromosome 5 (Macciardi et al, 1992; Hallmayer et al, 1992), and the expansion of unstable gene (Ross et al, 1993; Petronis et al, 1995; Sasaki & Kennedy, 1995). Reich (1995) reviewed three reports of linkage studies of bipolar genes (Berrettini et al, 1994; Straub et al, 1994; Pekkarinen et al, 1994) and suggested that the disorder might be caused by progressive intergeneration expansion of trinucleotide repeat sequences. This "anticipation" has already been found responsible for fragile X syndrome and Huntington's Chorea. In spite of the differences at this early stage, psychiatric geneticists were optimistic about what modern molecular genetics could bring to psychiatry in the near future:

> Over the coming years susceptibility genes for several psychiatric disorders will be identified. This will lead to dramatic improvements in the understanding of the pathophysiology of these disorders and will enable the development of more rational and specific therapies as well as the possibility of preventing illness developing in some susceptible individuals. Clinical psychiatry in the 21 st century is likely to be revolutionised by these developments. (Craddock, 1996)

> As we have seen, the inheritance of psychiatric disorders and behavioural variation is complex...However, recent methodological developments together with the knowledge and technology provided by the Human Genome Project mean that we can now be reasonably confident that at least some of the genes contributing to common psychiatric disorders will be identified by the end of the first decade of the 21 st century. It also seems likely that recently commenced work on the molecular genetics of behavioural traits and dimensions will begin to identify some of the genes involved in areas such as personality and cognitive abilities. (Owen & McGuffin, 1997)

Few psychiatrists nowadays would argue the total determinism of genetics. The more scientists come to learn from familial studies and molecular genetics, the more they will appreciate the complexity of the problems involved. The nature-nurture paradigms are not antagonistic to each other (Goldsmith, 1993; Wachs, 1993) and their effects cannot be separated. (Plomin, 1990; Rutter & Plomin, 1997)

Limitations

While genetics received given an impetus from the latest DNA techniques of genetic engineering, further testing of more specific pathogenic hypotheses is required particularly into how the defective gene(s) act metabolically, and the interplay with environmental factors. Technological advances in molecular biology do not diminish the importance of the classical approach. This is due partly to the valuable contribution of familial studies which have constantly improved methodologically, and partly to the genetic heterogeneity that molecular genetic studies revealed. In spite of the occasional excitement brought by the success of single gene probes (as in the case of Huntington's disease), and the gradual discovery of physical maps, genetic maps and the complete nucleotide sequence of human chromosomes (Lander, 1996; Schuler et al, 1996), development simply has not reached a stage where polygenic relations are clear. The mode of inheritance remains obscure and apart from the crude notion that environmental factors play a role, there is little clue as to how genetic and environmental factors interplay. At the moment, environmental influence can only be inferred by the part unexplained by genetics. It is hoped that when the genome projects launched in different countries yield most information about the susceptible genes, the role played by the environment will become clearer than it is now.

While the technology and the theoretical framework of the gene mechanism have been improving, many of the prevalent concepts of genetics remain problematic and biased. Wexler (1992) noted that newspaper headlines conveyed powerful but often biased concepts about genetic disease and many commonly held ideas about genetic disease in the family are just not right. Rutter and Plomin (1997) gave a detailed account of these misconceptions which include wrongful ideas 1) of genetics: genetics means single abnormal genes; genes associated with disease must be bad; 2) between genetic and environmental influence: genetic effects are unaffected by environmental intervention; genetic effects are determinative; and high heritability renders environmenal intervention ineffective; 3) of the implications of genetics: heritability estimates have a "true" fixed value for each trait; differences of heritability between populations will also be genetically determined; "bad" genes justify eugenic programmes and termination of pregnancy; genetic screening of the general population will be useful and gene therapy will be widely applicable. These misconceptions were challenged with empirical and clinical evidence and the authors presented a balanced view on what is meant by genetics and what benefit it could bring to clinical psychiatry. The genetic-environmental debate is expected to continue in a more rational way, and discussion is likely to be more disorder-specific instead of treating both genetic influence and environmental influence each as homogenous. One example of this trend is the deliberation of genetic-environmental interaction in aggressivity and conduct disorders (Cadoret et al, 1997).

Compared to the development of molecular genetics, studies of environmental influence over the course or cause of psychiatric disorders are less developed. One major problem is that environmental influence is not universal. It is always person-specific. Another problem is that some environmental factors may indeed be pre-set by genetics, and it is equally possible that social or environmental situation can lead to genetic consequences. These two examples are but illustrations that genetic and environmental influence are less separable than they first appeared to be.

Family studies have indicated strongly the existence of a genetic element in the etiology of certain types of disorder. The degree of risk seems to correlate highly with the degree of genetic relatedness. This conclusion from various studies stands scrutiny even when tighter and operationally more well defined diagnostic criteria are applied in new or replicated studies. Conventional genetic concern clusters around twins, adoptees, and offspring of disordered parents, and has constantly improved with more powerful statistical methods like path analysis and latent model fitting. However, it has largely neglected the fact that all first degree relationships are the result of mating between spouses, and there has rarely been adequate attention directed to the mating pattern itself.

The choice of partner contains major familial influence in the form of communication, degree of love and care, cultural practice, and overall quality of life within the family. The picture given by genetic studies will not be complete without an understanding of how choice of partner has contributed genetically to the generally higher risk of disorders found in first degree relatives. Judged from the almost equally high risk of MZ twins and offspring of dual mating, the genetic implication of dual mating must receive at least as much attention as twin studies. To re-establish an emphasis on spouses is potentially significant in two ways. First, whether people with disorder or predisposition to disorder tend to choose a partner with disorder (or predisposition) has implications, as a psychosocial situation may have genetic consequences, which in turn has implications for the prevention and treatment of mental illness. Second, if like chooses like, it is important to find out whether the assortment tendency is illness-specific (Negri et al, 1981; Merikangas & Spiker, 1982), or generally applicable to mental illness as a whole (Merikangas, 1982). This will enable further studies to gear their efforts and resources more effectively into this new area of concern.

Evolutionary Forces

Natural Selection & Sexual Selection

More than a century ago, Darwin noted the tremendous struggle of the animal world for survival and reproduction. Most animal species are capable of reproducing at a much quicker rate than the regeneration of resources; they have to compete for scarce resources, and consequently competition poses constraints on their population expansion. In the respect of survival and reproduction, all species are found to be selfish, and the competition for resources for these two purposes is not limited to tooth and claw, but also involves strategies helped by the variation of different traits. Some species have developed physical weapons while some display strange behaviours or physical traits to attract a mate. It is under this condition of natural selection that there exist different mating strategies between the sexes. Darwin (1859) distinguished two types of sexual selection [mating strategy]. The species have to compete with members of the same sex - intrasexual selection, and to make choices about which members of the opposite sex they prefer to mate with - epigamic selection. The extent of these two types of sexual selection obviously varies according to different species as an indirect result of sex ratio and the mortality rate of the sexes.

In other words, natural selection exerts evolutionary pressure on the species which must differentiate in sexual selection in order to have the best possible survival and reproduction rate through the selection of mates. It is generally accepted by biologists that mate selection according to certain characteristics (voice, attractiveness, dominance etc.) would preserve better gene(s) which in turn determine such traits of mating. The choice of a stronger and more dominant male would be more likely to carry on genes of this trait to the next generation. On the other hand, not only do attractive women appear to have higher reproductive success, they are also more likely to trade attractiveness for male paternal care and investment. In general, men and women adopt different mating strategies. While women try to ensure more resources are invested in each single potential offspring, men seek to maximise the number of offspring possible, through polygyny (Betzig, 1986), monogamy and adultery (Fisher, 1992).

Universalities of Human Mating Evolutionists believe that human beings are also under similar evolutionary pressure that the animal world faces (Trivers, 1985) and support for this view is drawn from some universalities of human mating regardless of different cultures.

Firstly, some forms of marriage exist in all cultures. Daly & Wilson (1979) surveyed more than 800 human cultures and found that although most cultures permit polygyny, most people mate monogamously, and the marital bond is universal even in the case of polyandry. These universal phenomena, together with differences in selection criteria for partners between the sexes, are unlikely to be explained satisfactorily by the sex roles and sex-related values prescribed by the norms of human society. There is also some evidence that, like most of the animal species, dominance in men enhances male attractiveness (Sadalla & Fausal, 1980; Sadalla et al, 1987).

Secondly, as other species, men are more inclined to engage in sex than are women. Men are more willing to sleep with someone in the absence of love, but women are more likely to do it to someone they love (Hinde, 1984). Men are more sexually eager irrespective of culture (Messenger, 1971; Marshall, 1971), and are more likely to view sex and intimacy as separate (Lewis et al, 1978). More men than women volunteered for experiments on erotica (Kenrick et al, 1980). This is in line with the suggestion that men seek more experience with erotica (Kinsey et al, 1953; Shepher & Reisman, 1985), and are over-represented in every category of sexual deviation (Davison & Neale, 1982). However, this male promiscuity is different from that of other mammalian species in that it is moderated by factors like heavier paternal investment, the bond between the pair, and in most western culture the homogamous nature of human mate selection. Although the male is more inclined to sexual relationships, the female chooses mates who are more likely to invest in their offspring. This, together with the bond and the modern homogamous marriage system, reduces the possibility of investing resources endlessly outside the mating pairs.

Thirdly, hormonal influence plays a role in the heterosexual relationship. Testosterone is connected with sexual interest in both sexes (Svare & Kinsley, 1987), dominant behaviour (Mazur & Lamb, 1980), and is involved in several stages of the relationship (Kenrick & Trost, 1987). That fact that men produce more testosterone than women may explain why men make more sexual advances than women. Although hormones do not seem to affect whom one will choose to be one's partner, it sets in motion the need for the search of mate and sexual advances once a member of the opposite sex is initially approached.

Parental Investment and Sexual Selection

In both the animal and the human world women invest more in the bearing and the care of offspring than men. This partly explains the "female choice" in mating despite the fact that women possesses less socio-economic resources than male does. In most circumstances, women are highly discriminating in the choice of mates even if competition is keen among women for dominant men. In contrast, men are generally less choosy than women since they have less to lose from an ill-chosen mating.

Human offspring take a much longer period than the offspring of any other species to grow before they become independent. This means that the human infant requires more care and resources for nurture. Hence we should explore that a female would tend to choose a man who could offer a better nurturing environment to the offspring whereas a male would value those traits that signal health and reproductive power, like beauty and youth (Buss & Barnes, 1986). The differential parental investment perspective may explain why men and women differ in their mate selection criteria.

From an alternative perspective, differential parental investment can be seen as a form of exchange of resources. Evolutionists do not see the exchange process as equity based. It is not regarded as a conscious calculative process, but as being compelled by the powerful and irresistible evolutionary forces for reproduction. Exchange theorists put heterosexual exchange into a wider framework of exchange of all human relationship, but evolutionists take the exchange between different sexes as a distinct exchange relationships. The purpose of exchange is distinct - reproduction; the process of exchange is distinct - differential sexual selection; and part of the commodities exchanged is also distinct - the presence of emotional commodities alongside other resources involved in the exchange. Love is a special resource that one values only when it comes from certain intimates, and is mainly exchanged in kind (Foa & Foa, 1980). Therefore, the exchange relationship between heterosexual partners is fundamentally different from other human exchange relationships.

The Reproductive Exchange Model Kenrick & Trost (1987) first proposed a five-stage model of relationship formation: stimulus search, establishing contact, trait assessment, establishing physical intimacy, and bond maintenance. These five stages should not be regarded as a general model for the analysis of a relationship, but are specific to the heterosexual reproduc-tive relationship. Two years later (1989), the two authors used the same perspective to analyse two of the major issues which had not received consistent support - sex difference in relation to age and resources of the chosen partners.

In the first issue, they disagreed that the general trend for the female to choose a slightly older male was due to social homogamy or the prevalent normative value in any given society. When they re-analysed an earlier dataset (Kenrick & Keefe, 1989) with male-female dimension, and different age (from lonely-hearts advertisements), there was a clear difference of preferred age between male and female advertisers. Apart from the confirmation that women tended to seek older men and men to seek younger women, the most interesting finding was perhaps that, irrespective of their own advancing age, men of all age groups except those in their sixties preferred women within reproductive years. It was argued that such a difference did not reflect in itself the value of youth in women, but the fact that women have a shorter period of reproductive years than men do. If the argument is that of social homogamy or similarity, similarity of age between couples should occur to all age groups.

In the second issue, different aspects of sexual preference were found. Notably, economic and related resources of men were much preferred by women as a criterion for a long-term partner (Buss & Barnes, 1986) and in meeting strangers, dominant men were found to be more sexually attractive to women than others (Sadalla et al, 1987). This difference was apparently due to situational factors and the difference in the nature of duration of partnership. To overcome this methodological problem of one single state at a time, Kenrick and colleagues (1990) separated respondents into groups according to four different stages: date, sexual relations, date steadily, and marry. Female subjects showed a consistent and gradual rise in the expected lowest acceptable intelligence of mates from the first to the fourth stage. It appeared that the more intimate and confiding the relationship progressed into, the more women expected on the quality of their partners. On the other hand, men had a sharp fall of expectation in the second stage - sexual relations, indicating a less demanding attitude towards those with whom they had had sex. This particular pattern would have been concealed if there had been no separate analysis by stages of relationship. When the stages progressed, the difference of expectations between the two sexes narrowed. Although women seemed to be more "choosy" over the status-linked variables, men were nearly as selective as women when considering requirements for a long-term partner. Clearly the differential selection criteria were due to an interaction effect between gender and courtship stages.

The evolutionary perspective has gradually shifted its emphasis from natural selection and the preservation of the fitness gene to the adaptedness of the species. The former tends to explain better the situation of a normal population than of psychiatric patients. People with a genetic problem have a better chance of survival if the problem gene is "diluted" in the offspring (i.e. by choosing a partner who does not have the problem). This contradicts the ample findings that there is initial assortment between people suffering from varying degrees and types of mental health problems. The latter solve this dilemma by suggesting adaptive functions of intimate relationships which not only apply to a normal population, but also to a treated population. Psychiatric sufferers, known for their limited resources and social ability, are less resourceful in exploring and sustaining confiding relationships. Partnership in itself is both joyful and stressful. By choosing someone who is "similar" to oneself, people feel accepted and understood. The immediate social environment is made familiar, predictable and supportive.

Critique

The evolutionary perspective is essentially a bio-social model. It attempts to incorporate and integrate different fields of knowledge, including biology, personality and social psychology, sociology, and anthropology, and it is most noticeable for its contribution to an emerging field called evolutionary psychology (Kenrick & Trost, 1993, 1997; Kenrick, 1994; Simpson & Kenrick, 1997). The psychosocial determinants of partnership can now be given new meanings. Irrational romantic love, economic exchange and social stratification of partnership are blended for the preservation of species and better adaptedness. The split between psychological and sociological perspectives is no longer necessary.

This perspective has given a clearer picture of how biological and social variables interplay. A psychosocial phenomenon like choice of mate can be of biological origin; biological reproduction can be constrained by social variables like the marriage system; the choice of partner may affect the selection of genes for traits that facilitate successful mating. Although psychologists have repeatedly been aware of the genetic implications of assortative mating, it is the evolutionists who provide clues of how a gene of traits might be involved.

Among all perspectives reviewed, the evolutionary approach is the most recent and the one that is most able to absorb and reinterpret findings from different perspectives. The implicit assumption that all intimate heterosexual relationships are for reproductive purpose, however, is not compatible with the fact that some people deliberately enter into a marriage with an agreement not to have children (Veevers, 1980; Callan, 1983). In reality, there are so many situations that couples are forced to reconsider the need for having children, like instability of marital relationship, overwhelming financial burden and anticipated lack of time to care for the children. Given the limited resources available or the particular situation of the couple, survival is preferred to reproduction.

Conclusion

Evolution occurs both from within and without. The internal process is slow and the preservation of adaptive genes through natural selection has originally been designed by nature to modify genetic make-up through years if not hundreds of years. Balance was maintained through the extinction and survival of adaptive genes and traits. But now, with the latest DNA technology, genes could be manipulated, and to a certain degree corrected. The internal change has been speeded up, and possibilities of recovery or amelioration are being created for an illness that was once been irreversible or resistant to treatment. In the years ahead, there will be achievements from the human genome project and the various gene studies that are taking place in many countries. New technology brings about new situations and new dilemmas that have not been faced before. In contrast to the new fascination of genetic engineering, courtship and mating remain one of the oldest concerns in human society. Psychological, social, economic, and environmental forces continue to exert an influence over one's choice of partner.

In the next chapter, various ethical issues in relation to psychiatry will be examined, especially the dilemma that comes as part and parcel of the many new situations that psychiatric patients have to face.

4 Key Ethical Issues

Modern technological advances in health care have brought about new issues and dilemmas well beyond solution at the technical level. New situations emerge as a result of changing personal, technical, and organizational contexts. Euthanasia, abortion, informed consent and rationing of health resources are some of the issues most interesting to academics and the public. Compared to other medical specialisms, psychiatric practice appears initially to be least concerned with medical technology and to give a less contentious outlook. This, however, is certainly not the case when the nature of psychiatry is closely examined. The problems and difficulties facing mental health professionals are embedded in, and perhaps inherent in its very nature. These concerns have been well aware of in major texts (Bloch and Chodoff, 1991; Dyer, 1996).

Since debates often begin with values and philosophical principles, we will first examine the Hippocratic Oath, which has frequently been interpreted either as supporting or refuting argument. In discussing the relevance of the Oath to mental health practice we shall inevitably come to discuss some of the more fundamental issues with people suffering from mental ill health, including autonomy, competence and consent to treatment. It is argued that mental health practice faces dilemmas far more complicated than do other practices, involving questions as fundamental as the definition of mental illness and personhood. In the last part of this chapter and in the light of these earlier discussions, and given their relevancy and importance to this study, the often neglected ethical issues of genetic engineering and human reproduction in relation to mate selection will be discussed.

Hippocratic Tradition

The fourth Century B.C. Hippocratic Oath has been regarded as the original source of practice principles for medical practitioners, and it has often served as a basis for the development of codes of ethics for major medical associations. Apart from the concern of the obligation of members of the Hippocratic community towards their teachers and their family, the major part of the text is devoted to issues of the doctor-patient relationship. In modern terms, they are concerns and instructions about responsibility and good work: "I will apply dietetic measure for the benefit of the sick according to my ability and judgement"; no harm principle: "I will keep them from harm and injustice"; euthanasia: "I will neither give a deadly drug to anybody if asked for it, nor will I take a suggestion to this effect"; abortion: "I will not give to a woman an abortive remedy"; patient's benefit first: "Whatever houses I may visit, I will come for the benefit of the sick, remaining free of all intentional injustice, of all mischief and in particular of sexual relations with both female and male persons, be they free or slaves"; confidentiality: "What I may see or hear in the course of the treatment or even outside of the treatment in regard to the life of men, which on no account one must spread abroad, I will keep to myself holding such things shameful to be spoken about."

Most criticisms of the Hippocratic code turn on its insufficiency. The Hippocratic Oath is too ancient to cope with new demands (Altman, 1979); it deals with the doctor's obligation, not the patient's rights (Chapman, 1984). Others (Dyer, 1996) defended it and suggested it has a "legitimacy both in providing guidelines to practitioners and in helping patients know what to expect" (p.37). Of course what is stated in the Oath is far less than what it is not stated, especially in view of modern medical technological advances and the unimaginable complexities faced by the medical profession at group, organization and national levels. It is, however, the intent and concept behind these codes and the conflicts between them which interest us most, because it is exactly these conflicts that are at the centre of the problem and difficulties encountered by mental health practice. Criticisms of being out-dated or too simplistic do not interest either practitioners or theorists and provide little clues as to the understanding of the complicated picture which emerges from where medicine, psychology, and philosophy intersect.

Dilemmas in Paternalistic Care

The first and foremost concern of the Hippocratic Oath is about the paternalistic nature of medicine. The code presupposes that doctors know what is best for the patient and can carry it out for the patient with their professional judgement and skills. This virtue throughout medical history has been very much accepted because patients know that they are patients and they trust the intent, knowledge and skill of the doctor to tackle his health problems. But this trust is not taken for granted in psychiatry. From time to time, there are disturbing reports of political dissidents being detained as mental patients (Szasz, 1994b) and of the co-operation of psychiatrists with military governments in the torturing of political prisoners. Not only are these illustrations of how the trust and good intentions expected of psychiatrists can be abused when no measures are taken to safeguard the rights of patients, but also they demonstrate the increasingly complicated interests of the parties involved. What used to be a matter purely between doctor and patient now involves "society", the "common good", or the "state" and the morality of the profession cannot be decontextualised from the morality of the polity.

Paternalism in psychiatric care, as is the case with all medical specialisms, is closely tied to the obligation to care; but in the case of psychiatry, the boundary of care extends from physical health to behaviour that would have an adverse effect on patients and others. Hospitalization of involuntary patients and treatment against their own will are examples of the multi-faceted roles of psychiatrists. No other medical specialism has equivalent statutory power over its patients. The state has charged psychiatrists with the duty to care not only for patients but also others. Detention against one's own will is either based on the benefit of the patient or the protection of others (HMSO, 1983). This power is often criticised as an infringement of civil liberty (Szasz, 1986; 1994a; 1994b). At a conceptual level, the opposing arguments represent two major philosophical approaches to the matter. The first approach, often named Utilitarian, involves maximising the happiness of the greatest number. The second approach treats individual basic rights as ultimate and absolute, and therefore inalienable.

Utilitarian approach takes the patient's interest as the first consideration but final decision rests on the maximum aggregate utility of all parties. Therefore, the criticism that the patient's interest is the one and the only consideration, or, conversely, that the patient's personal benefit can be forsaken because incarceration of the patient will bring even bigger happiness to others are not justified. True utilitarians give no favourable weighting to the parties involved and it is the greatest pleasure or benefit to all parties that they pursue. Then problems arise as to whose benefit is to be considered: the family, the general public, or the institution that the psychiatrist represents? What is meant by benefit or happiness? Who is going to prevent damage caused in the name of benefit, and how? Above all, even if there is consensus as to harm and benefit, what is to be done when one person's happiness is another person's misery? Eventually utilitarians have to concede that although there is no difference in the nature of benefit for all people, there is an order or priority of consideration according to the peculiar situation. The order can be an answer to conflicting interest, but again the basis for the ordering can be problematic. Many case studies and lawsuits have demonstrated that utility is not a concept that can be applied in such a straightforward way as one may think (Veatch, 1997).

The current situation requires psychiatric professionals, mainly psychiatrists, psychiatric social workers and psychiatric nurses to make a medical decision on a course of action. These professions form their knowledge base variously from biological medicine, psychology, and social theory. Other medical specialism can claim expertise in a given human organ, or a piece of body machinery: the eye, the bone, the ear, the kidney, the foot, but psychiatrist deals with what he / she can call the "brain". What the "brain" normally refers to, however, are actually thoughts and feelings, and indeed mind and soul. The mechanistic determinism of cause-effect relations in natural science is borrowed to analyze the part of the person with which other professionals like psychologists and philosophers are also very much concerned.

While psychiatry has a legitimate claim on psychiatric patients, this does not make the specialism a monopoly provider of expertise on all problems of the mind. Whereas other specialisms have specific technologies to help diagnose and treat, psychiatric diagnosis is based primarily on conversation. Surgical operation or impact work on the physical brain like ECT are either abandoned or rarely resorted to. The concept of disease and illness is even more problematic. A medical or disease model presumes a known or reasonably suspected biological cause leading to certain physical manifestations in terms of symptoms or syndrome, and treatment is accordingly geared at removing the cause or reducing the severity of suffering brought about by the symptoms.

Judged on these criteria, it is not surprising that psychiatric diagnoses except those with a clear organic base, are based on a classification system which is in fact a systematic collection of symptoms. One is diagnosed as having "depression" because one has the sign of depression. The lack of conceptual specificity on the responsible disease entity makes it particularly difficult to claim the same level of technology, certainty and expertise which characterise other medical specialisms. With increasingly precise diagnostic classification systems like ICD-10 or DSM-IV, fewer patients are told of different diagnoses, but the problem remains in the limited information that these diagnoses tell or imply on the treatment. This embarrassing position of psychiatry can clearly be felt by Michels' (1991) remark:

> Psychiatry today worries about itself, its definition, its identity, its boundaries. There are many reasons for psychiatry's dysphoria – its scientific basis isn't what it would like, its public acceptance is tenuous, its status among related professions is dubious, its patients are often less than grateful, its claim on resources, both public and private, is probably questioned more than that of any other medical specialty, and its practitioners are more likely to find themselves in television comedies, New Yorker cartoons, or murder mysteries than on the list of prospective Nobel laureates for the coming year. (p.61)

The utilitarian approach to the problem depends heavily on its ability to observe and judge without much contention what is actually the problem, and the corresponding resolution. Neither the technology nor the nature of psychiatry seems to support such certainty and consensus.

The rights-based approach regards certain rights as basic and inalienable, like freedom from compulsory treatment or detention in mental hospital against one's will. The normal doctor-patient relationship is an interpersonal contract freely entered into by the patient and from which the patient may withdraw at will. The contractual relationship simply does not exist in any case of involuntary hospitalization. Proponents of this approach draw their support from historical evidence, and the ethics of "personhood", of which respect and autonomy, are integral parts:

Except the very young and the severely cognitively impaired, all human beings are rational, autonomous, and capable of making choices the way they like even though it may not fit in with our or certain groups' conception of a good and worthy life. It is this respect for autonomy and liberty that allows people's life different from one another. This respect has clearly been reflected in pledges of patient rights by hospital authorities in different countries.

Prior to the assumption of right is the presumption of personhood. It is commonly held that their clinical condition of any kind does not make psychiatric patients any less human than people with other kinds of problem. There are, however, two legitimate exceptions to this principle. First, in a situation where the whole personhood or an integral part of it, like competence for decision making, is lost, at least temporarily. To hospitalise someone for one's own good is morally not admissible, but if one "cannot" decide for oneself, there is a need for proxy decision making. This is especially true when psychotic patients relapse and lost their ability and consistency to decide for themselves. Second, if it can be proved that psychiatric patients are at a state of "sub-personhood" where principles of basic worth and respect will not be enjoyed to the full extent, like the case of children, there is no ethical problem of treating them not with their full right. This is particularly when an autonomous choice would damage one's or other's autonomy now or in the future.

Lindley (1988) cogently argued that the ability to choose is not equivalent to autonomy because current choice is necessarily but not sufficiently autonomous. While a value like autonomy is defended as intrinsic, it does not mean that value shall triumph at all time. He demonstrated that when autonomy clashes with avoidance of pain – the other side of pleasure, autonomy will be reduced to achieve the avoidance of pain. In other words, it is justifiable to restrict one's autonomy to prevent one from suffering considerable pain. Autonomy is not of binary discrete nature, and in real life, people are experiencing restriction on it either by themselves or by others in a natural and acceptable way, often in the hoping of obtaining something more valuable to themselves. Basically, Lindley supported earlier work (Culver & Gert, 1982; Gert & Culver, 1997) that not all paternalistic action damage a person's liberty of action, but he went further to argue that restriction of autonomy is allowed when it is done out of respect for one's autonomy.

There are situations where one's autonomy is not regarded as absolute. This is especially true when the patient is acting on false or distorted information, under undue influence or simply does not have the competence to make an autonomous choice. Delusions, hallucinations, and biased perception often lead those in confused state unable to make either a consistent choice or one that is for the interest of the decision maker. It is common that schizophrenic patients even in a relatively stable and non-confused state, do not have the awareness of being ill, and hence they do not regard treatment as necessary. Thomasma (1983) took autonomy not only as basic right to be respected, but also as a goal to be achieved. When an illness makes it impossible for the patient to decide for himself / herself, treatment that acts to restore one's ability for decision making is therefore justified.

The Right to Treatment and the Right to Refuse

Hospitalization

Rights often conflict. On one hand, the liberty of the individual (Veatch, 1981) and the right to refuse treatment have to be respected. On the other, individuals have the right to treatment for their own benefit, even though they may not be aware of the benefit that the treatment might bring to them. One has the right to be hospitalised and treated even when one does not consent to it at the time.

It might be thought that voluntary hospitalization is less contentious, but in fact it is not. Voluntary hospitalization enables patients to seek help more promptly and be more psychologically prepared to fall in line with the treatment received, and patients do not have to go through the legal procedures that might impair trust in a doctor-patient relationship. However if voluntary hospitalisation is not purely an administrative category that patients submit to in fear of being committed involuntarily, "voluntary consent" must be given. Voluntary consent means that 1) one has been given adequate and sufficient information; 2) one has the competence to make a decision and; 3) the decision is made voluntarily. This consenting capacity, as distinct from what is usually meant in a legal context, does not require full information, certainty about the expected result, and a full appreciation of rights, obligations and implications of the decision. As psychiatrists are not legal experts and the disclosure of non-medical information like the implication of social stigma was not an accepted practice among other medical specialties, Hoge (1994), refuses to accept a "strong" model of consent which requires more extensive disclosure of information including clinical problems, anticipated treatment, alternative treatment, legal rights, and discharge procedures. Rather, a less demanding - "weak" model was proposed.

Poythress et al. (1996) compared voluntary and involuntary psychiatric admissions, and supported Hoge's different model of consenting capacity. Almost two-thirds of the voluntary group (63.3%) showed impairment in understanding the disclosed information compared to nearly half of the involuntary group (46.7%). Contrary to the common notion that voluntary admissions are related to less problematic clinical condition, they found that clinical variables had relatively less influence on understanding voluntary admission. This raised the concern that psychiatric patients now have less protection than other kinds of patients if there is not the need to observe the full comparable model of consent. It is not uncommon to hear accusations that some psychiatrists resort to threats of compulsion in the absence of consent, rather than patiently explaining the need for in-patient care.

Levine et al. (1994) found that older patients who are admitted voluntarily have more difficulty than younger patients with questions about obtaining release and legal assistance. Billick et al. (1996) proposed a 15-item questionnaire to evaluate a patient's competency to consent to voluntary hospitalisation and succeeded in obtaining satisfactory parallel validity with a number of psychiatric rating scales and a vocabulary test. Such tests focus more on patient recognition than patient memory and recall (Poythress et al, 1996). Other studies also deliberated on the need for more comprehensive considerations (Lippert & Stewart, 1988; Kaplan & Price, 1989). By adopting criteria different from normal cognitive tests, these studies yielded a greater proportion and a more positive look of "competent" patients (Appelbaum, & Grisso, 1988; Grisso & Appelbaum, 1995; Slobogin, 1996; Stefan, 1996; Winick, 1996).

In some cases, commitment to hospital is based primarily on the will to protect of others. In this sense, hospital care serves as a control of behaviour and is justified on medical (not criminal) grounds, and entails medical treatment but in a secure setting. This conveys particular interpretation of the cause and extent of personal responsibility, and the appropriate treatment for the behaviour. Like other social control when the patient is considered acting not by "himself / herself", responsibility is denied but autonomy forfeited, with the consequence that one is no longer considered fit to choose what is best to oneself.

While in the light of the danger of abuse, involuntary detention for treatment usually has time limits, many patients have mental health problems which require long term managed care either in institutions or in the community. The lengthy period in which autonomy is diminished in such situations raises various ethical dilemmas, including the charge of creating dependence and incompetence (Dickenson, 1997). It is perhaps even more complicated when involuntarily committed mental patients are actually competent to refuse medication. Binder and McNiel (1991) found that in the hearings held for involuntarily committed patients, one-seventh of them fall into this category.

There are rather few studies on how patients perceive involuntary admission or treatment. Naber et al. (1996) interviewed 40 psychiatric patients, more than three-quarters of whom were diagnosed schizophrenic, on the restrospective experience of involuntary neuroleptic injection or restraint. Almost half the subjects rated the measures as necessary or positive though they also expressed a number of reservations. Allegedly fear and powerlessness were the predominant feelings in the face of coercion. Although the focus of concern of that study was on the determinants of acceptance or refusal of treatment, it did remind one of the importance of practical arrangements in hospital care that could have resulted in better subjective respect and well-being. Kjellin and colleagues (1997) compared a voluntary admission group with a compulsory admission group. Although more of the former group reported improvement and benefits, both groups demonstrated that the more one perceived oneself as being respected for autonomy (apart from admission), the more improvement one reported on one's mental health. This appears to support the thesis that compulsory admission in itself does not necessarily deprive one of a sense of respect and autonomy. It is rather the procedure and care upon and after admission that influences the subjective evaluation of autonomy, respect and perceived benefits.

Treatment and Consent

Treatment is only possible when the patient submits or is made to submit to it. Therefore it is not the form of treatment (voluntary or involuntary), but rather the ground for being made to submit that is called into question. Patients of other kinds have the right to refuse treatment even to the point where life is jeopardised, and no proxy decision is needed so long as the patient is considered competent to make such a decision. In most cases, commitment to hospital is based primarily on the benefit of the patient. This is justified when it can be established that 1) commitment increases the chance of improvement of mental state, which is beneficial to the patient; 2) non-commitment does greater harm than losing freedom for some time. By the latter (a Utilitarian principle), it does not deny the infringement of liberty but places it in the context of a value system which defines when infringement is tolerable and when not. Currently and unfortunately, the resolution of this ethical problem rests on a medical decision where consensus might not be taken for granted. The psychiatric judgement is based on a knowledge system which has far less certainty and determinism than other natural sciences.

Even in the case of those who gave consent to treatment, it is not without problems. By informed consent, we mean that the decision to consent was made on the basis of reasonable knowledge of courses, consequences and available alternatives. While most medical professionals would not have forsaken the procedure required for informed consent because of its implication for both the treatment of the patient and the professional code, Manning and Gaul (1997) observe that health care service providers give greater priority to warding off possible accusations and charges than to the participation of patients. Informed choice is not just an administrative duty, but an ethical principle which entails the active involvement of the patient in his / her healing process (Fisher, 1997). Abramovitch and colleagues (1993) found only four out of seventeen geriatric subjects considered competent to consent to mental capacity assessments, in spite of the impression held by the assessor that they all provided informed consent. Accordingly, there always exists the risk of assuming consent, yet without having it in reality.

It is true that most acute patients admitted for psychiatric treatment were incompetent to consent (Hoffman & Srinvasan, 1992), but it is equally true that there are also other factors, like low education level and older age (Cournos, 1993) and insensitive practice, limiting the true spirit of consent to treatment.

Role of Psychiatrists

Psychiatrists are more than clinicians. No matter where we stand on the line about aligning the profession with the government or the military, it is certainly correct to point out the distinct duty of the psychiatrist to care beyond medicine. One example is combat psychiatry for the armed forces since World War II and its increasing role in modern warfare. Assisting soldiers, though in quite a different way, to kill and better cope in the battlefield entails tremendous ethical conflicts between convictions held for civilian and military, and has been poorly understood and discussed (Artiss, 1997). It is mostly the caring and gate keeping role that was discussed and made the psychiatrist's role vastly different from other medical specialisms. On one hand psychiatrists and other psychiatric professionals have to decide for the benefit of the individual, and on the other to take into account the possible risk and harm to both the individual and others. The dual role of power and professional responsibility has seldom perhaps, been brought into such sharp focus as in psychiatry (Rinella & Gerstein, 1994; Appelbaum, 1997).

Another example is about the controversies in forensic psychiatry. The duty to report domestic violence and other unlawful deeds may jeopardise the working relationship by breaking confidentiality in early stages and discourage people to come for the care that they need. Psychiatrists are constantly faced with the dilemmas of mandatory reporting of domestic violence (Hyman et al, 1995) and of child abuse (Adler, 1995). Forensic psychiatrists have been continuously asked to predict the dangerousness although most legal systems concern only behaviours rather than the inclination to behave. To restrict one's freedom on the basis of prediction is ethically unsound, unless it can be established that such a prediction is made in acceptable confidence. A few studies reveal that the accuracy of prediction of assaultiveness increased with the duration of follow-up (Zeiss et al, 1996) and that command hallucinations is a good predictor of self-harm (Klasper et al, 1996). However, the problem remains as to what level of confidence is acceptable.

It is assumed that psychiatrists know what is best for the patient, and this assumption is loosely linked to their medical knowledge and expertise in psychopathology. The public seldom query the competence of the psychiatrist in understanding of the pathology, accuracy of classification and diagnosis, giving the right kind of treatment, and making predictions about any possible danger caused to or by the patient. In brief, the psychiatrist has the power of deciding the timing and the form of treatment, and this power ranges from clear medical reasons to purely behavioural concerns. The diagnostic tools and diagnoses made are indeed systematic and carefully classified descriptions of symptoms, and the diagnosis alone does not necessarily add new knowledge or understanding about the etiology of the illness. The limitation of the present knowledge system and the tremendous impact of such a classification has been well noted (Beauchamp & Childress, 1982; Brody and Engelhardt, 1987; Greenberg & Bailey, 1994). It is on this ground that psychiatrists have to make assessments and predictions. There is some evidence that mental health professionals are over-concerned with rules and regulations even in cases with a remote risk of a lawsuit (Bernet, 1995).

Nowadays, there is still evidence that psychiatry is being applied to control political dissidents in a number of countries. Mental patients in industralised countries on the other hand face constraints of a different kind. In a context of increasing in-patient costs and managerial demand for more cost-effective psychiatric services, the psychiatric professions are given new roles to determine the mode of service delivery and who deserves what services. This dual and often conflicting role is of concern more to expert clinicians than inexperienced medical staff. Health care reforms have created large number of clinicians-turned managers who have to take care of the interest of not only individual patients, but also the department and organization in which they work. In societies where health care delivery relies partly or heavily on private companies, such dilemmas are more apparent.

> The pressures on psychiatrists and all other physicians to limit care are becoming difficult to resist. Professional ethics provide one of the few

> constraints on managed care machinery in the marketplace arena. The preoccupation of managed care with profits has led to insensitivity to medical ethics and a lack of interest in it. This problem has prompted a proposal to develop ethics for managed care that include a balancing of medical ethics and economics. ...Managed care marketplace considerations provide no incentive to treat high-cost, severely ill patients who have limited financial resources. (Weinstock & Leong, 1996)

Roles are but sets of expectations reflecting how one's function is perceived and demanded, as a result of the particular political, social and economic context. To draw a line between what is appropriate and what is not is difficult and perhaps impossible, but at least the roles of psychiatric professions should not be taken for granted as simply clinically-based without discussion and reflection.

Gene Ethics

The Promises

The Human Genome Project of United States which started in 1990 attempted to map the entire genetic make-up of human beings. Progress is well ahead of schedule (Collins, 1995), and it is expected that in the first half decade of the 21 century the sequence of the entire three billion base pairs of genes will be marked. By then, when the entire data set is available, pathologists will unlock the genetic code for diseases, and the public will be able to check against the risk of all major diseases. Corresponding treatment (pharmaceutical or non-pharmaceutical) will be directed to the sufferers more effectively. It is not necessary, however, to wait for the final revelation to taste the fruit of the work. The susceptible gene has been identified for cystic fibrosis (Kerem et al, 1989; Welsh et al, 1995) and breast cancer (Miki et al, 1994) and it would not take long for major polygenic psychoses to be similarly identified.

Parallel to the concern for technical breakthrough is the concern about social life, which is likely to be affected tremendously by this new knowledge. As an integral part, the genome project also involves an evaluation of the major ethical, legal, and social implications. These areas are considered so important that, in a recent report, it has been recommended need for the participation of non-professionals at a policy level:

> There is no doubt that policy issues must be considered at a level that not only permits but encourages full participation by all interested parties, including

> concerned members of the public, professional societies, government regulatory agencies, and the research community. In other words, policy development must occur at a level that provides a public forum for discussion of these critical issues and not only permits but encourages the active participation of all of the stakeholders to formulate and implement policy. (National Institute of Health, 1998)

Diagnostic Screening

Diagnostic screening at a presymptomatic stage has enabled early detection of diseases. The screening has already been made available for a few diseases affected by single gene defects. The IVF technique, the culture of cells and the DNA sequencing of the genome altogether require teams of experts and will not be publicly available upon a patient's request. Universal screening is costly and not an effective means of case finding. As in the case of Hungtington's Disease and cystic fibrosis, many people who have undergone such screening are not at risk of currently having the disease or of having an offspring who would suffer from the disease. For the few who have been rightly identified as either carriers or potential patients, there is a legitimate ethical debate as to what good it is to find out some diseases that are incurable and inescapable. Although there is consensus that predisposition testing should be limited to diseases that are treatable or preventable, no one is certain how this principle will be implemented and monitored as more and more diagnostic tools are developed. Psychological fear would have been easily aroused especially when misconception about heredity is common not only among the general public but also the medical professions. Patients in question are likely to experience distress, stigma and discrimination when their rights are not properly protected (Billings et al, 1992; Greely, 1992). It is perfectly sensible for some to have the right to know, and some others the right not to know.

Like government hospitals and laboratories, biotechnology companies in some countries have also developed relevant diagnostic tools and made the laboratory service available in the market for certain diseases including Cooley's anemia, Mediterranean anemia, familial breast/ovarian cancer, Duchenne/Becker muscular dystrophy, Fragile-X syndrome, hemophilia A, Huntington's disease, sickle cell anemia and Charcot-Marie-Tooth disease. One only needs to pay and send back the cell sample (usually blood cells) for the tests. The service has been criticised for its reliability problem. False positive often causes unnecessary psychological distress whereas false negative reduces caution to guard one's own health.

Genetic screening is particularly valuable at the perinatal period. Genetic tests give accurate diagnoses of certain genetic defects of the fetus and the mother has more valid information to choose whether such a pregnancy should be stopped. For the anti-abortionist, geneticists become the accomplices to abortion. There will be less contention when there exists more serious form of genetic defects. It can be problematic in how mothers and medical professionals decide what defects are serious enough to seek an abortion when perinatal genetic screening is available for a wide range of genetic defects of which some are more detrimental than others. With the aid of in vitro fertilization (IVF) and ex vivo technology, prenatal screening is also possible. Grifo and colleagues (1998) have recently reported the successful outcome of preimplantation diagnosis for genetically transmitted diseases with embryos obtained by in vitro fertilization from patient groups in the third day of its life. Sixteen embryos were diagnosed as being unaffected, of them 37.5% implanted. This recent development has been possible to avoid the complicated legal, moral, and psychological impact on both patient and possibly doctor. However, when most parents or more exactly to-be parents accept prenatal screening to prevent having offspring with serious genetic defects, there will be new sets of ethical problems with regard to reproductive choice and eugenics.

Current psychiatric diagnosis, as we have previously shown, is based mainly on classifications of symptomatology. If most psychiatric disorders have a genetic basis and could be correctly identified genetically, there will be a new ethical dilemma. Most psychiatric illnesses do not develop identifiable symptoms until early adulthood (schizophrenia and affective disorders) or late adulthood (dementia). Many parents would be anxious to know whether their own children were at risk of developing a severe psychiatric disorder like schizophrenia or mania. Successful identification of a genetic defect at an early age would mean that some parents would have to bear the distress and fear throughout the years with no certainty for that the illness would ever develop (Wexler, 1992). Should children being tested have the right to refuse the genetic screening on themselves? Should parents be allowed for a genetic screening on their children even though there are no observable symptoms? Should parents have the right not to refer their children for genetic screening even if they were considered to be in a high risk group? These are all difficult questions that deserve discussion and reflection.

The Use of Genetic Data

Genetic data are highly personal but their usage has a range of broader purposes. As genes affect not only the individuals, but their families, there is a legitimate ethical concern as to whether personal "defected" gene data should be communicated to one's spouse, siblings and other family members. The effect, whether the results are supportive or rejecting, could have a chain-effect. Outside the family, employers would be eager to shed their medical costs and keep a workforce that is more productive and less disturbed by various diseases. Data could be used for recruitment, promotion, and dismissal of the genetically disadvantaged in the organization. This would obviously be discriminatory, but should the data be kept only for the purpose of self-knowledge, the benefits would obviously be very limited, leaving the workforce virtually intact even with the understanding of new effective ways to improve it. Insurance companies are also keen to know the genetic risk of the insurers so that the high risk group would either be excluded or have to pay a much higher premium. Protection of the genetic data of the insured varies in different parts of the world, but current discussions are limited mostly to the United States and European countries (Knoppers & Chadwick, 1994).

Reilly and Page (1998) discussed the worrying trend of genetic data banks that contain information on huge number of persons. Among the various data sources, the DNA database on convicted criminals in UK is growing fast and will soon include thirty percent of all males aged thirty or more. The US counterpart follows the practice of collective DNA fingerprinting and will eventually reach a comparable size. Pharmaceutical companies also hold vast amounts of genetic information and there is also ethical concern over the commodification of genetic data. It has been reported that more than ten million newborn babies are screened annually in the West for certain genetic diseases and metabolism disorders. Intrusion of privacy, misuse of information and over policing are but a few examples of possible abuse of the DNA data. There were once even fears that sooner or later mankind would be stratified socially according to the defective genes, with people carrying certain defective genes classified as a new subhuman species with restricted welfare and political rights.

Gene Therapy and Eugenics

Since approved gene therapy was applied successfully to Little Ashanti who was suffering from severe combined immunodeficiency (SCID) in 1990, gene therapy has been on trial to about a hundred diseases, ranging from cancer to rheumatoid arthritis and AIDS (Anderson, 1995). The existing gene therapy techniques work on the somatic cell and aim at correcting a genetic defect by replacing the bad gene of certain cells or by inserting a corrective gene to exert the right effect. Ethicists seldom oppose somatic gene therapy because of its therapeutic effect and its inability to alter one's own and one's offspring's genetic constitution. The effect of the somatic gene therapy depends very much on the nature of the delivery system through which the corrective gene is installed, and how able the delivery system is in evading attack from the immune system. Existing delivery systems by microinjection, fusion or virus are often short-lived, low in transfer rate and suspicious to and weakened by the immune system. Injection of the right gene has to be repeated in order to prolong the effect. With the present state of the art, once a patient shows signs of improvement, gene therapy has to be kept on irrespective of the present and future cost because it would be unethical to withdraw a treatment which had been started. Gene therapy in utero is considered viable because a fetus of 12-14 weeks has been found unable to reject foreign tissue and cells (Patterson et al, in press). This will overcome the existing problem of rejection and re-action of our immune system to the corrective gene. Before this time, pregnancy is often a one-null question. Now there are going to be new considerations as the fetus can be operated on.

As with issues encountered in genetic screening, gene therapy also meets with the problem of equity. It would have taken some time for somatic cell gene therapy to become widely available to patients in need. Who is to decide which patients need what kind of treatment, be it genetic or non-genetic? Certainly, not all major diseases will be tackled, because increasingly stringent health care resources would mean some loss of opportunity in the treatment and service for those diseases not chosen. Should more resources should be used for gene therapy, the result of which is mixed at the moment, or be allocated to non-genetic treatment of diseases with proven results? Many other diseases are simply left untreated because of lack of resources.

Germ-line therapy works at a different level. When genes are corrected and put back to the fertilised egg or the fetus, the correct DNA sequence will replicate itself and remove the risk and harm presented by the defective gene. Also the corrected gene make-up will be passed on to offspring, breaking the hit of heredity between generations. Germ-line therapy in theory should be more thorough and effective, but has not been officially approved for a number of reasons. Firstly, any mistakes in gene would be transmitted to the descendants, but finding the degree of safety and risk of this gene therapy which is acceptable to both geneticists and ethicists is difficult. Secondly, it is about the level of technology achieved. So far, genetic technology even for somatic cell gene therapy is not mature enough for massive curing. None of the hundred cystic fibrosis patients on trial somatic cell therapy has been cured, and perhaps more extensive trials and further improvement in technique are required before there is certain proof of success. For germ-line therapy in animals, success is also questionable. The microinjection of DNA often harms the egg and in experiment conditions, only about 2% of the surviving eggs carried the gene. It is technically difficult to ensure the injected DNA would migrate to the right position of the chromosome. It is difficult to imagine how this technique could be used in humans who have only limited eggs in a period of time, and how scientists would handle the failures which are supposed to outnumber the successes. Because the technology is at such an elementary stage, Anderson (1992) does not think the attempt to improve the human species is in any way a real threat or promise.

To prevent potential abuses of genetic engineering, scientists repeatedly called for vigilance and the need for the public to be well-informed:

> The only way to ensure that history does not repeat itself is for the scientific and medical communities to remain constantly vigilant for abuses of genetics. (Watson et al, 1990)

> Eugenic genetic engineering , on the other hand, is purely theoretical ....The best insurance against possible abuse is a well-informed public. (Anderson, 1992)

> Our society went into the age of nuclear energy blindly, and we went into the age of DDT and other pesticides blindly. But we cannot afford to go into the age of genetic engineering blindly. Instead we must move into this exciting new era with an awareness that gene therapy can be used for evil as well as for good. As we reap the benefits of this technology, we must remember its pitfalls and remain vigilant. (Anderson, 1995)

This optimistic view of vigilance and public accountability by medical professionals is not shared by some analysts. Proctor (1989) found that the racial hygiene programmes to clear up the Jews, the poor, and the "feeble-minded" under the Nazis had been carried out with the support and co-operation of many health professionals, including psychiatrists. Dyck (1997) looked back into history and found medical staff closely involved in atrocities and abuses not only in Germany, but also in other European countries and the United States, based on their commitment to improving human welfare. Now there is again revived interest among scientists to achieve the removal of some genetic diseases, and, one step further, improvements of the human species in general (Carlson, 1987; Roll-Hanssen, 1988). Professional conscience is not a guarantee, and it is uncertain whether it ever will be. Spallone (1989) traced how eugenics in the past became a means of creating or exacerbating racial, sexual and class prejudice, and how the Eugenics Society, transformed into modern guise, was still able to draw on the enthusiasm of many scientists including some prominent figures in genetic studies. Many scientists refused to discuss eugenics because technology has not yet reached that stage, but the intention and interest are always there.

It is doubtful whether the professional community and the state would allow genocide to recur in the name of eugenics. However, eugenics may breed or reinforce prejudice and racism. There have been complaints from Jewish organizations that research on "Jewish" genetic diseases might reinforce and fuel racial prejudice. This worry is not without ground. Well-intentioned genetic studies among segregated groups could result in prejudice by others. In discussing genetics and racism, Reilly and Page recently observe:

> Racism and ethnic strife may be the most dangerous and intractable problems in the modern world. From ethnic cleansing in Bosnia to hatchet killings in Rwanda, humans see all too eager to view their neighbours as inferior or evil. Is it possible that deeper knowledge about the human genome and its diversity could help resolve this problem? Or could such knowledge reinforce racial stereotypes and worsen the situation? (Reilly & Page, 1998, p.17)

The role of government has changed considerably and the racial issue has become more delicate and difficult to handle than hitherto for most governments. Irrespective of how much the state itself was involved in the development and promotion of genetic engineering, most countries in the West are so concerned about the potential misuse of genetic studies that different procedural and legal regulations have been adopted for the aspects of protecting privacy, preventing unnecessary harm and regulating experimentation on human embryos. However, on the other side of the world, where human resources and burdens become increasingly a concern for emerging countries, ideas about eugenics are being translated into practices and policies affecting the lives of many. Chan (1992) described how social policy in Singapore attempted to preserve elitism by encouraging fertility among educated women, and inducing sterilization among less educated women. Instead of helping women to achieve a better education, the control of human reproduction legitimated and rationalised social inequalities. Debates broke out in the 18th International Congress of Genetics held in Beijing in relation to the 1994 Infant Health Law. The law in question forbade individuals with certain genetic diseases to marry unless they agreed to be sterilised or to take long-term contraceptive measures. Although officials pointed out that the law had never been enforced, critics remained to be convinced (Normile, 1998). Abortion of fetuses with abnormalities has been the usual practice and even normal "extra" fetuses become victims of the birth control policy.

On the one hand, the involvement of private enterprises and non-state organizations in the development of genetic engineering did reduce the state's role in direct participation. But on the other hand, it will not take long for business entities to envisage a lucrative future in gene correction, be it for disease or general improvement purposes. Choice of sex of babies is currently available, and further possibilities of genetic improvement will emerge along with the gene projects. At a time when technology is available for some parents to improve on what their own genes would produce, of course at a cost, there will be resentment among those who cannot afford it and those who are denied the opportunity. Currently, companies have invested huge sums in genetic research. The patenting of results and techniques raise another ethical issue because while access to the technology is inevitably restricted, its effect on the lives of many people is profound. Do these intellectual properties actually belong to mankind rather than the ones who discovered them? How much more than the cost should the state pay the patent owner? Is it ethical on the part of the state to transfer part or most of such cost to patients? These questions may appear to be too distant at the moment, but many critics are skeptical about current reliance on market forces in the development of genetic research and concerned about its implications (Paul, 1994).

Reproductive Choice and Genetic Counselling

Genetic technology has expanded choices among human reproduction. Choice may mean choosing to keep or abort the fetus, and choosing to conceive and receive genetic structure from a third party, and choosing to mate with another person who does not possess the same defective gene. The first choice is especially pertinent as one has to admit that most diseases and disabilities found genetically among fetus are incurable. The choice in that case might appear likely to be abortion. At least in the foreseeable future, debates over abortion will be closely tied to the human genome project and the application of more advanced diagnostic tools. It is expected that gene technology will catalyse decisionmaking for the new form of abandonment – abortion. Successful germ-line therapy in the future might provide another viable alternative to abortion, but in view of the massive number of abortions that take place every day, a comparatively small amount of high-cost germ-line therapy would appear not cost-effective. For those who try to avoid transmitting problem genes from the partner, third-party sperm banks are a viable alternative. Sperm banks and IVF technology provide an alternative to conceiving without increasing the genetic risk of phenotype. The inclusion of a genetic structure not belonging to the partner and not having concerned genetic defects has reversed the process of natural selection but still speeds up the inhibition or removal of the gene in question. However, unless the use of third-party sperms takes place on a massive scale, the genetic structure of the population will not be altered. Ethical problems arise as to whose offspring one is, and when the third-party sperms are used not because of infertility of the original sperms, but for the avoidance of possible genetic damage.

The final choice is not usually available to patients because it is virtually impossible to have a preliminary screening on a prospective partner before entering into an intimate relationship, unless the effect of the defective gene is so debilitating that the party concerned is extremely conscientious in selecting a partner who does not have the same genetic defect. Such a deliberate mating strategy has been adopted by some Jewish groups to prevent the occurence of known phenotype in their offsprings. The strategy simply involves the dilution or decentralization of problem genes, but obviously against the matrimonial vow of commitment to whatever kind of adversities – "in sickness and in health". At least we are beginning to understand that environmental factors like this situational consideration potentially have genetic consequences. The interference by government varies according to different countries. It is a source of major ethical concern when reproductive choice is taken over by government, and when abortion is regarded as the only acceptable or permissible choice.

Genetic counselling services are currently provided to couples in countries where genetic screening is available. In most countries the service is not been available to all citizens, and is usually available only upon referral or patient request. The role of the counsellor is very much determined by the infrastructure of the service. When genetic counsellors work more for the health care policy directed by the state than for their own professional code, patients will easily be seduced into believing the keeping of the pregnancy is not for the benefit of the mother and the country. An international survey of genetic counsellors found that all Chinese respondents and a few Western respondents thought that the purpose of genetic counselling was to reduce bad genes in the population (Normile,

1998). Quaid (1994) documented how a female patient, distressed by genetic counselling, struggled eventually to become a founder of the National Hereditary Disease Foundation. Although her contribution to and achievement of the self-help movement is exceptional, her personal experience with genetic counselling may be less so.

Conclusion

There are overwhelming ethical issues in psychiatry. Some issues, like the right to treatment and to refuse treatment, proxy decision making, and basic human rights like autonomy and competence, are common to patients of other medical conditions. Some other issues are particular to the psychiatric profession, like involuntary admission and compulsory treatment. The dilemmas often go into as deeply as the philosophical base of personhood, and the inherent problems of psychiatry. There are no easy answers to the questions, but it will be less confusing if a time dimension can be added to psychiatric disorders. Psychiatric disorders are not homogenous, and nor are they static. The residual abilities of patients vary along the time-line. The time and kind of treatment and other social variables differ from one patient to another. It seems difficult and theoretically insufficient to uphold a definite ethical perspective at all times for psychiatry. The issues are so difficult that some have tried to handle them in terms of process instead of outcome. Procedural fairness has been claimed to safeguard the patient's rights. This spirit is evident in the suggestion of employing a team decision to arrive at inter-subjectivity and consensus on what is best for the patient concerned. It is the author's opinion that unless, proved otherwise, psychiatric patients should best be regarded as capable of making autonomous decisions for themselves, and that marginalisation and abuses should always be discouraged.

Different arguments derive from different theoretical premises, and the questions will not be answered satisfactorily by the fast-growing technology in human genetics. In contrast, while genetic engineering and the unveiling of the human DNA sequence are revolutionalizing our understanding of the etiology and manifestation of many diseases including psychiatric disorders, these innovations have also brought about new situations and dilemmas which have never been faced before. Among them are new issues and concerns for the privacy in relation to genetic information, genetic screening, reproductive choice and eugenics. Hope and despair coexist when diagnostic screening techniques are well ahead of corrective gene therapy. Geneticists and ethicists have constantly been reminding others about the unfolding benefits and harms to mankind by genetic engineering.

While we may be fascinated by what genetic engineering can bring to science and the well-being of mankind, it has to be reiterated that gene technology does not change the genetic structure of the population. It is the mating and its subsequent reproduction that determine the genetic structure of the population. Behind mating, the forces are social, psychological, and situational in nature, propelling the evolution of social adaptedness notwithstanding what happens molecularly inside. Choosing a partner of not having the same defective gene is clearly an example of how social situations can have genetic consequences. In this study, we approached the issue from the social end. Did psychiatric sufferers tend to choose a partner with similar phenotype or characteristics? If so, what could this have meant for their adaptedness and survival?

5 Methodology and Measurement

Sampling Frame

In order to test these hypotheses, two groups of patients: schizophrenic patients, and depressed patients will be compared. Each patient of the first group is diagnosed as suffering from schizophrenia whereas each patient of the second group is diagnosed as suffering from neurotic depression by ICD-9 diagnostic criteria. Both groups of patients are living currently with a partner (legitimately married or cohabiting). The reasons for choosing the two diagnostic groups are that schizophrenia is most affected by heredity whereas depression is found to significantly related to one's social and marital situations (Brown & Harris, 1978; Bebbington, 1987). The schizophrenia group also represent those are suffered from more severe forms of psychiatric illness and have more enduring debilitating effects. Neurotic depression is a less severe form of psychiatric illness and has less disabling consequences.

Finding a sufficient number of schizophrenic patients who are still with a partner was not easy. The (chosen) hospital records indicated that only twenty two potential schizophrenic subjects were of married or cohabiting marital status.

Unfortunately, sixty four per cent of them had major life events like divorce, separation, moving house, and unstable mental state that made them unavailable or unsuitable for the study. Of the remaining eight suitable cases, one refused to participate. In order to increase the size of schizophrenic sample, the help from Making Space (the former North West Schizophrenic Fellowship) was elicited. The proportion of treated schizophrenic subjects with a partner (6.6%) was found quite similar to that of the hospital. Consequently, of the fifty five members contacted, one third expressed their willingness to participate in this study.

It was decided that a sample should first be drawn from the schizophrenic patients and then to find matched subjects from the depressed group, based on sex and age.[1] The twenty-five schizophrenic subjects were matched on sex and to the nearest possible age to married depressed patients. In case of refusal, consecutive cases were picked up from the list. Of the sixty six depressed patients and their spouses that the worker contacted, thirty five per cent experienced major life events (i.e. divorce, separation, bereavement, or moving house) that rendered them unsuitable for the study. The successful return rate for this group is thirty eight per cent. The summaries are shown in Table 5.1.

Table 5.1 Breakdown of Case Finding Figures

	unsuitable because of changed life situations	refused by patient or the spouse	Completed pair of cases [a]	total cases contacted
SCH Group				
hospital setting	14 (63.6%)	1 (45.5%)	7 (31.8%)	22 (100%)
community setting	2 (3.6%)	35 [b] (63.6%)	18 (32.7%)	55 (100%)
DEP Group				
hospital setting	23 (34.8%)	18 (27.3%)	25 (37.9%)	66 (100%)

[a] patient and spouse are counted as one pair of cases. There are twenty five pairs of couples and therefore fifty individual cases in each group.

[b] those who did not respond were assumed not interested in the study. It is likely that the high percentage may actually consist those who had become unsuitable because of changed life situations.

The schizophrenic group participated in this study represents a significant proportion of treated schizophrenic patients who remain in a marriage or confiding / cohabiting relationship. The schizophrenic group in this study nevertheless may be different from schizophrenics who do not remain in a marriage or long term relationship and different from other psychotic

---

[1] The matching of length of marriage is impossible because there is no prior information as to this variable.

patients. If that is the case, the matched comparison group of depressed patients may not be at all representing the depressed patients who are still in a marriage, but of a rather more selected group. As a consequence, it will be easier to make generalisations about the schizophrenic group than it will be about the depressed group who have been matched to the schizophrenia sample.

When the average age of the participants is compared with that of the non-participants of the chosen hospital who indicated "married" status, the participants are about two years older. The differences are not statistically significant – see Table 5.2. Therefore, it is believed that for those who indicated "married" status, the participants are not very different from the non-participants in age.

Table 5.2 Age of Selected and Overall Cases

	Participants Mean (SD)	Non-participants of the (chosen) hospital [a] Mean (SD)
The Schizophrenic Patients	45.1 (9.7) N=25	42.8 (11.2) N=28
The Depressed Patients	46.6 (9.3) N=25	43.0 (11.8) N=214

[a] Those patients who indicated married status when they first contacted the hospital. The figure included those who could not be contacted and refused to take part in the present study. The non-participants of the second group also included a small number of patients suffered from other neurosis.

Sampling-Related Issues

For the method of consecutive pick-up to yield a randomised sample, the sample population that fits the research criteria must be reasonably large, with no obvious problem of replacement. Clearly it is not the case of this study. The cases found are not randomised, but judging from the small numbers of potential cases that may fit the criterion of being married and still upholding the marriage, the cases picked up are believed to represent a significant proportion of the treated group (particularly the schizophrenic group).

Another issue is the nature of marriages among selected subjects. As expected, all pairs are of one male and one female. It will not be valid for whatever findings to be generalised to other confiding relationships beyond heterosexual homogamy. The subjects selected are mostly white British, and therefore it seems inappropriate to extend any argument to either cross-cultural marriages or marriages of other different cultures or races.

The scope of marriages under concern is in every way a very limited one, but the research focus and boundary is clear and appropriate for a small research project like this. It is especially important to restrict the concern to certain issues in order not to loose the focus. The fact is that most dimensions of mate selection among psychiatric patients are virtually not explored and this study is hopefully just a start of its kind.

Administering Procedure

A letter was sent to the patients who appeared to meet the research criteria. Those who did not refuse were given the questionnaires and return envelopes. Instructions were printed on the questionnaire and repeated again when the worker handed over the questionnaire to the respondents: (1) there is no right or wrong answer; (2) it is essential for the couples to answer the questionnaire booklet separately without discussing with each other; (3) the data will be treated as confidential.

Help was arranged in situations where the respondents felt they needed it. A small number of older patients or their spouses required help in filling the questionnaire. Twenty-eight per cent of the couples in the schizophrenic group and twelve per cent of the couples in the depressed group completed their questionnaires together with the research worker. There were no follow-up contacts except in a few cases of unclear answers or un-completed sections.

Statistical Procedure

The returned questionnaires were coded and analysed with the use of SPSS. Different statistical tests and procedures are employed, depending on the nature and coding of the variables. Percentage listing and non-parametric tests are used for some nominal / ranked data variables. Chi square test is used for two-way cross-tabulation where required. Kappa's coefficient is calculated for within-pair agreement for some variables like illegal drug usage and drinking.

However, Kappa's test of agreement is not considered an optimal measurement for this study. Essentially, it gives a ratio which is a function of exact agreement of categorical data, not the proximity of answers. It works perfectly well for dichotomised variables where the disagreement falls precisely into adjacent cells. It is also suitable for variables where answers are nominal and bear no relationship with one another. For categorical variables where less exact agreement is expected than "near" agreement, the Kappa's figure fails to indicate such a relationship. It will be fair to remark that Kappa's test does try to indicate the agreement between two situations, but only succeeds in detecting the most typical and observable part of the agreement, not the direction of agreement, nor the more subtle form of close agreement.

The parametric T-Test has frequently been used for the test of mean score differences, even in the analysis where only the patients or their spouses were compared by diagnostic groups. Although in the latter situation the sample size is below the common threshold of "thirty", parametric T-Test is still used because of the belief that the schizophrenic group sample represents to a large extent the population of those schizophrenic patients who are in an intimate relationship. Paired-sample T-Test is used when either the patient groups, the spouse groups, or each pair of couples in the same diagnostic group are compared. Independent T-Test is also used where grouping by sex (e.g. male patients and spouses in the schizophrenic group compared with female patients and spouses in the same group) does not yield a matched comparison.

Where parametric T-Test appears to be strictly inapplicable, Mann-Whitney U Test will be used when the categories of the data can be ranked. If the variable concerned is only nominal in nature, Kruskal-Wallis Test is sometimes used to check if there is any difference in the distribution of the groups.

When the means of more than two variables are concerned, analysis of variance will be carried out to ascertain the main effects (diagnostic groupings, sex, patient-spouse status) and different level of interaction effect. In such analyses, the sample size will become bigger (N=100) to justify a parametric test instead of a non-parametric test.

Principal component factor analysis is also used in several occasions where it is believed that there are common factor(s) underlying the variables. Unless otherwise stated, varimax rotation is employed, with the assumption of independent factors and error terms. Discriminant analysis is also used in some occasions to predict membership. Wilk criterion is used throughout.

Where regression is used for a simple path model, it is assumed from the individual hypotheses tested that certain causal relationships exit between the variables. Each path coefficient has to pass the T-test, and the regression formula as a whole has to meet the F test criteria that the beta coefficients as a whole are significantly different from the zero assumption. It is also assumed that the error terms of each dependent variables are not correlated. Standardised beta is reported instead of the raw score beta in order to avoid the problem of interpretation because of the difference in the measurement unit. All the variables involved except one are ratio data. That is the binary variable of whether or not first met through medical setting. A one indicates "yes", and a null indicates "no". The nature of the variables justified its use.

Measurement

Apart from questions asking about demography, the questionnaire consists of four main sections: a self-designed questionnaire for courtship and marriage, the General Health Questionnaire (GHQ-28), the Eysenck Personality Questionnaire, and Maclean's 46 statement on psychiatric illness and psychiatric patients. Most questions of the section on courtship and marriage are of five-point scale; 1 indicating the least agreement and 5 indicating the most. This section was designed by the research worker because there were no existing inventories that appeared to serve the purposes of the present study. The GHQ is widely regarded as a valid inventory for the measuring of minor psychiatric disturbances (Ballinger, 1975; Kirk & Saunders, 1979; Corser & Philip, 1978; Ballinger et al, 1985). In the present study, the GHQ-28 version (Goldberg & Hillier, 1979) is used because of its sub-scale structure of four different symptomatological dimensions. The EPQ is a valid inventory for the measuring of personality traits (Campbell & Reynolds, 1982; Gong, 1984; Kozeny, 1984, 1986, Wilson & Doolabh, 1992). The ninety-item EPQ is preferred to its earlier version for its inclusion of a new variable - psychoticism or "tough-mindedness". Later versions like Eysenck Personality Scales (Eysenck & Eysenck, 1985) were not used because the addiction and criminality scales are not relevant to the present study. Maclean's 46 statement questionnaire is less popular, but is included for the measurement of two social opinion scales: the Social Distance Scale and the Social Sympathy Scale.

Conclusion

The method involved in this study is certainly not perfect, in view of the complicated nature of the area being researched, the mounting difficulties in case-finding, and the limited resources available to the researcher. The questionnaire itself has not undergone vigorous piloting process, and the wordings of the items (e.g. Are you hard to "get" ?) are often open for subjective interpretation by the respondents. However, one must remember that it is the subjective opinion of the respondents that the study is trying to elicit. Some may doubt seriously the ability of psychiatric patients to answer questionnaire, and also fear the undue influence due to the lack of awareness of being ill, but these questions are common not only to this particular study, but also to all other research works which require psychiatric patients to give answers or responses. In fact it is believed that the social data from the patients are less likely to be contaminated than the clinical data elicited from them because social data appear to have less connection with their state of mental health.

6 Results

Reliability

The questionnaire used in this study can broadly be divided into five main parts: socio-demographic data, courtship and marriage data, a General Health Questionnaire (GHQ-28), an Eysenck Personality Questionnaire (EPQ), and an opinion survey including two attitude scales, the Social Sympathy Scale and the Social Distance Scale. The present study as a whole are asking one to provide information and opinions on issues that are related to oneself and one's partner, and therefore one's role can be regarded as a combination of self-reporting (giving own information) and informant (giving partner's information). Self-reporting, in the case of psychiatric patients, has long been accepted as a reliable source of information for social and clinical assessment. Patients, in most cases, do give reliable reports of their own symptoms and social situations (Kenny & Bounous, 1961; Berger et al, 1963), although what the patient reported reflects one's own perception and frame of reference which are subject to the influence of more severe symptoms (Kosa et al, 1967; Polich, 1982; Watson et al, 1984b). Since most patient subjects of the present study are not on active treatment regime, there is no reason to believe that they gave unreliable information. Anthony (1989) showed that there were no qualitative differences between self-reporting and the information from informants (people other than the patient) and both type of information can be taken as valid measures of the patient's clinical and social situations.

The first specific question raised will probably be how reliable is it for couples to report courtship and marriage data that might be from ten or fifteen years ago. It has to be admitted that longitudinal testing at each and every stage of the courtship and marriage would be ideal, but certainly costly and intrusive. Besides, given the very limited number of schizophrenic patients still with a partner, this approach would likely end up with only a few cases. To ask them to report information retrospectively is not the best method, from the view of experimental design. The real concern is actually whether the subjects will distort or misrepresent the information intentionally or unintentionally. Apart from the person's own motivation and the environmental influence that he is subject to, the extent of "true report" also depends on how and what the questions are being asked in the questionnaire. In this study, only impressions are asked for, not the minute details of interaction, nor the delicate inner feelings. The questions are straight-forward, like "Was he / she hard to get ?", "Were you hard to get", and in case where there would be different possible answers, a number of alternatives are requested: "can you name three things that your partner was most attractive to you at that time?"; " Can you give three reasons why you married your current partner?" In fact the respondents were told that there are no right or wrong answers and they were allowed to leave a question unanswered if they could not think of any answer.

The initial draft of the questionnaire has been tested by a group of five couples married for different lengths of time, who were friends of the researcher in a local church. They were all interviewed later with regard to the ease of answering the questionnaire, and clarity of the questions asked. Four couples managed to complete the questionnaire in 30-40 minutes, and an older couple took about 50 minutes. Some of them raised the concern that some items (item 18, 61, 64) of EPQ were unnecessary because they thought that nobody would answer "no". They had no problem with GHQ at all. As far as the social attitude inventory was concerned, two partici-pants expressed that they found it hard to answer about a few items (item 37, 38, 39) because "it depends" on the situations. A participant did not answer the two questions about his parents because they passed away when he was small. Two participants answered the questions of previous situations with current situations. They all found the part on courtship and marriage interesting and almost all said they had not answered a questionnaire of this kind. They all agreed that they should be allowed to call on the researcher for help in case they had any problem with the questionnaire. Finally although they answered the questionnaire separately, they were all very eager to know the answers of their spouses, particularly the part on how their spouses thought they were.

As a result of these feedbacks, the two questions about one's parents were further reviewed. Not only are there situations that render the question not applicable (i.e. early separation from parents, parents died at the time of one's courtship), but also that the parents may hold different opinions between themselves. However, these situations should not be common. It was finally decided that these two questions remained unchanged, but the participants should be told to write "NA" or "not applicable" to whatever question that does not seem to fit them. Each of these two questions was positioned as the last question of the page so that there is space for participants to write their comments in case they need. The layout of section on courtship and marriage is also rearranged with big bold heading stating the timing of the questions that followed. The order of the courtship and marriage questions are also rearranged to avoid confusions, but all standard inventories are used in their original wordings in spite of the feedbacks on certain items. To reduce possible problems due to illiteracy, and misinterpretation on ambiguous terms, the researcher made himself available to all participants. They could choose to go through the questionnaire with the researcher, or to call on him whenever they have any problems in answering the questionnaire. If the participants preferred to being inter-viewed, they would be interviewed separately. The researcher has made a set of answer cards with big prints for the interviewee to choose. The researcher also had to spell out clearly to the participants that they were not to answer the questionnaire in the presence of their partner, and one should not try to make the other answer favourably about oneself. Otherwise, their answers would not be helpful to this study. Nevertheless, they could discuss their answers only after they have completed the questionnaire.

To test out the final draft of the questionnaire, the first five couples of the schizophrenic group were interviewed separately with the questionnaire. With the help of answer cards, all but one patient can answer quite smoothly. That patient did not feel well and consistently could not answer many questions. To avoid situations like this, all questionnaires returned were checked by the researcher. When there were a few questions unanswered, follow-up contact will be made with the respondents to make sure it is not due to unstable mental health condition.

Because of the lack of financial support for the project, this study did not involve other research workers. Since this study did not require subjective scale-rating by the researcher, there was no attempt to establish inter-rater reliability.

Internal Consistency of the Standard Inventories

Given the cross-sectional nature and the small number of cases in this study, only the internal consistency reliability (Cronbach's Alpha) is calculated. If the coefficient of this sample differs significantly from the ones collected in the manuals, it will then be reasonable to doubt if it is reliable for them to be applied to this particular sample. As there is very little information available in the literature about the two social attitude scales used, it is expected that they may have relatively lower alpha level than other scales.

Table 6.1 Internal Consistency Reliability (N=100)

Personality Traits	Psychoticism	0.48
	Extroversion	0.86
	Neuroticism	0.91
	Social Naivety	0.80
Symptomatology	Somatic	0.85
	Anxiety & Insomnia	0.89
	Social Dysfunction	0.89
	Severe Depression	0.90
Attitudes	Social Sympathy	0.46
	Social Distance	0.69

It is clear from Table 6.1 that the GHQ sub-scales and EPQ sub-scales except Psychoticism are at 0.8 level or above. The low Alpha level of Psychoticism is mainly due to the unstable scoring of the P dimension (high scores in some items, but low in some others within the same sub-scale) among patient subjects. According to Eysenck and Eysenck (1975), in fact the alpha coefficient of the P scale was between 0.68 (female normals) and 0.77 (female prisoners) - the lowest among all sub-scales. This study gives a level of 0.48 for P scale and there can be two explanations. First, the patient subjects as a whole are mostly discharged patients, their clinical situations became less acute than when they received active treatment. This resulted in drop of scores in some items of psychoticism, but not all, producing a highly varied inter-correlation between the items. Secondly, the schizophrenic patients and the depressed patients scored differently for different items in the P scale, making a low correlation between the items for the test as a whole.

As expected, the two attitude scales have lower alpha coefficients compared to the other inventories. Firstly, one has to understand that social attitude scales are more likely to be subject to changes and are internally less stable than other domains like personality traits and symptomatology. Second, there might be problems due to the inherent structure of the scale itself. The principal component analysis of Maclean's 46 opinion statement actually yielded ten factors (if the threshold of 1.0 eigen value is taken). There would still be three general factors if the demarcation is drawn from the scree test. The three factors altogether only account for one third of the total variance. Seven out of the eight items on the Social Sympathy Scale fall into the first factor, but there are also nineteen other items exceeding a 0.3 factor loading. Five out of the seven items on the Social Distance Scale are also included in the second factor, but similar to the previous scale, it embraces far more items than the author originally proposed. It appears that the social attitudes that the two scales supposed to measure, are fluid in nature. It is likely that the Social Sympathy Scale may only be measuring part of the domain that it intends to measure.

Validity

Criterion-Related Validity

One of the ways to establish the validity is to relate the variables concerned with a criterion. The first part of questions on courtship and marriage included six items asking about different areas of satisfaction. It is predictable that the more satisfied one was reported to be with the current marriage, the more likely he would be to remain in the relationship, and therefore more likely to choose the same partner again if one has the choice now. A discriminant analysis reveals that the satisfaction with one's own role, and the role of one's partner pass the Wilk's stepwise requirement and can actually predict correctly 84% of whether they would like to choose the same partner again.

Another support for criterion validity concerns extroversion and the number of friends. Since extroversion denotes a person's outgoingness, it is natural that extroverts appear to be more sociable and introverts less motivated to make friends. If extroversion is by and large a stable personality trait which does not change much over time, we will expect a positive relationship between extroversion and the number of close friends. It is found in this study that the correlation between one's extroversion score and one's reported number of close friend before current marriage is 0.38, significant at .05 level.

The other indication concerns the use of the two established scales EPQ and GHQ to identify those who suffered from mental illness and those who did not. Since the clinical condition of the patient subjects is not controlled, and the lack of clinical information of their partners, the prediction is not expected to be as accurate as up to the 80 to 85% level. Nevertheless, there should be a recognisable relationship between the predicting and predicted variables.

Table 6.2 Prediction of Membership by Discriminant Analysis

Predicted Membership	Predicting Variable [b]	Correctly Classified cases	Correctly Classified non cases	Total correctly classified
Sufferer [a] (N=58); non-sufferer (N=42)	Extroversion, Neuroticism	81%	69%	76%
	Severe Depression	56.9%	73.8%	64%
Patient N=50); spouse (N=50)	Extroversion, Neuroticism	76%	68%	72%
	Somatic Symptoms, Anxiety & Insomnia, Severe Depression	58%	78%	68%

[a] Six spouses of the schizophrenic patients, and two spouses of the depressed patients also self-admitted as psychiatric sufferers.
[b] All sub-scales of EPQ and GHQ are included before it is selectively removed by Wilk's criteria.

All sub-scales of EPQ and GHQ are included before it is selectively removed by Wilk's criteria. Six spouses of the schizophrenic patients, and two spouses of the depressed patients also self-admitted as psychiatric sufferers.

As shown in Table 6.2, two slightly different criteria are used: sufferer status and patient status. The two differ in that the former is self-report and the latter is determined by the availability of a diagnosis. It is clear that the extroversion and neuroticism sub-scales of the EPQ have a rather high rate of correct classification of cases whereas the sub-scales of GHQ was more predictive of non-cases. Although the GHQ is commonly used as a screening tool, it gives an overall assessment of current mental state which is not diagnosis-specific. The schizophrenic patients had a lower score on extroversion while the neurotic depressive patient had a higher neuroticism, making these two sub-scales capable of differentiating the schizophrenic patients and neurotic depressive patients from their spouses.

Content-Validity

Another way to ascertain validity is to look into the correlation between different sets of variables. If the content is largely valid, there should be more significant correlations between similar variables within the same domain than with variables of a different domain.

The correlation matrix depicted in Table 6.3 consists of several different sets of variables. The first set of variables concern courtship and marriage. The premarital relationship capacity is a factor variable derived from the number of close friends before marriage, the number of marriage, and the length of current marriage – see Table 7.1 of the next chapter for details of the factor loadings). Acquaintance through medical setting is a binary variable indicating whether or not one first met one's partner through medical setting. The general satisfaction is a factor variable derived from six areas of current marital satisfaction (doing activities together, feeling close to each other, talking and sharing with each other, own role as husband / wife, partner's role as husband / wife, showing affection and concern). The factor variables are factor scores and other social variables apart from the binary variable are of a five-point scale: one indicating the least and 5 indicating the most.

The relationship capacity is found to be negatively but significantly correlated with acquaintance through medical setting ($r = -.32$, $p<.01$), and age at the time of this marriage ($r = -.53$, $p<.001$). It is very reasonable that subjects with greater capacity to relate to others were less likely to have partners met through medical setting (coding as 1 or 0), and were more likely to have the current marriage at an earlier age. On the other hand, the age at the time of this marriage is positively and significantly correlated with general satisfaction. This means that the older the subjects entered into current relationship, the more satisfied they are about the current relationship. It will be shown later in this chapter that this was not due to the experience gained from previous marriage since the majority of the subjects were married for the first time. Finally, within this set of variables, whether one would choose the partner again is found to be significantly correlated with the general satisfaction ($r=0.71$, $p<.001$) and overall attractiveness of partner at the time of courtship ($r=0.37$, $p<.001$). While it is appreciated that the more satisfied one feels in the current relationship, the more willing one will be to indicate that one would choose the same partner again if one had the choice, it is interesting that the more attractive the partner was reported to be, the more likely the partner was to indicate that they would choose the same partner again. As predicted, this set of variables do not have any significant correlation (positive or negative) with variables of other sets.

The second set of variables are the sub-scales of the GHQ-28. There are significant correlations within the sub-scales and with the N and L scales of EPQ, but not with any other variables of other domains. Neuroticism correlates significantly with somatic symptoms, anxiety & insomnia, social dysfunction, and severe depression where L correlates negatively and significantly, though to a lesser degree, with the social dysfunction and severe depression.

The third set of variables is about personality trait sub-scales among which N is significantly correlated with E ($r = -.37$, $p<.001$) and L ($r = -.27$, $p<.01$). The use of oblimin factor rotation by the author suggested that these sub-scales are not entirely independent from one another. The NE correlation is not very different from the author's -0.22 to -0.33 range (depending on the samples). It agrees with the common notion that nervous persons are more introvert, and less likely to be socially naive. The reason why P does not bear a strong relationship with other within-domain sub-scales will be discussed in more detail in the discussion. The L scale, instead of being used uncritically as a "Lie Scale", will be reinterpreted as a separate personality dimension relevant to the situations of the subjects of this study. This will also be dealt with later.

Finally, the two social attitude scales correlate significantly with each other, but have very minimal linear relationship with variables of any other domains. Overall, the patterns of inter- and intra-correlation are quite in agreement with our understanding of the variables. A complete substantiation of the claim of validity will require a replication of this study with a larger sample size.

Table 6.3 Pearson's Product-Moment Correlation Matrix of Variables

	V1	V2	V3	V4	V5	V6	SUA	SUB	SUC	SUD	P	E	N	L	SS	SD
V1	1															
V2	-0.32*	1														
V3	-0.53	-0.25	1													
V4	0.04	-0.02	-0.08	1												
V5	-0.07	-0.13	0.31*	0.23	1											
V6	0.01	-0.22	0.18	0.37	0.71	1										
SUA	0.19	0.06	-0.19	0.13	-0.13	-0.03	1									
SUB	0.25	-0.00	-0.21	0.09	-0.19	-0.01	0.80	1								
SUC	0.17	0.00	-0.17	0.20	-0.11	0.04	0.63	0.69	1							
SUD	0.14	0.02	-0.14	0.19	-0.09	0.07	0.64	0.74	0.67	1						
P	0.12	0.05	-0.01	0.11	-0.02	0.04	0.23	0.17	0.16	0.26	1					
E	0.12	-0.08	0.07	-0.08	0.01	-0.11	-0.18	-0.21	-0.23	-0.25	0.12	1				
N	0.04	-0.08	-0.19	0.17	-0.03	-0.04	0.59	0.58	0.44	0.51	0.01	-0.37	1			
L	-0.05	0.15	0.23	-0.03	0.19	0.06	-0.15	-0.18	-0.28	-0.28*	-0.11	-0.01	-0.27	1		
SS	-0.11	-0.24	0.03	-0.01	0.08	0.08	-0.13	-0.06	-0.11	-0.08	-0.18	-0.05	0.17	-0.19	1	
SD	0.02	-0.03	0.02	-0.09	0.07	0.12	0.03	-0.02	-0.02	0.01	0.05	0.03	0.04	-0.05	0.32*	1

* sig. at 0.1 level ;
___ sig. at 0.05 level

keys - Social variables: V1 = premarital relationship capacity, V2 = acquaintance through medical setting, V3 = age at this marriage, V4=overall attractiveness at the time of courtship, V5= general satisfaction factor, V6 = would choose the same

Background Information

Age of Subjects

Patient's sex and age were matched for both diagnostic groups to the nearest patient in the hospital records, and hence there was no significant difference between the two patients groups. The patients and spouses of the depressed group were about 1 year older than those of schizophrenic group. Only one spouse in the schizophrenic group was in his twenties. Most patients and spouses were in their thirties and forties (Table 6.4).

Table 6.4 Age Range and Mean Age by Patient / Spouse

	SCH Group		DEP Group	
	Patient (Ps)	Spouse (Ss)	Patient (Pn)	Spouse (Sn)
MEAN (yrs)	45.12	45.96	46.56	46.52
SD (yrs)	9.68	10.36	9.27	9.24
AGE RANGE (n)				
20 - 30 yrs		1		
31 - 40 yrs	7	8	7	9
41 - 50 yrs	8	9	9	9
51 - 60 yrs	8	5	7	5
61+ yrs	2	2	2	2
Total	25	25	25	25

When grouped by sexes, men were slightly older than women for both schizophrenic group and depressed group (Table 6.5). It is interesting to note that the age of the spouses in both groups was not controlled, but the pattern remains similarly for both diagnostic groups. Clear there was a sex difference in the preference of a younger or older partner irrespective of the kind of mental health problem one suffered. Men in general preferred a younger wife or women in general preferred an older man.

Table 6.5 Age Range and Mean Age by Sex

	SCH Group		DEP Group	
	Male (Ms)	Female (Fs)	Male (Mn)	Female (Fn)
MEAN (yrs)	46.76	44.78	47.84	45.24
SD (yrs)	10.78	9.05	9.12	9.2
AGE RANGE (n)				
20 - 30 yrs	1			
31 - 40 yrs	7	10	8	6
41 - 50 yrs	11	8	6	10
51 - 60 yrs	5	5	8	7
61+ yrs	1	2	3	2
Total	25	25	25	25

Significantly high correlations were found between the age of patients and spouses for both groups of patients, but even stronger correlations were found between sexes for both groups (Table 6.6). This was due to the fact that husbands in both groups tended to have wives slightly younger (2.5 years) than themselves. This assortment of age between couples was in line with the normal population.

The age of the spouses was not controlled, but there was no significant difference in age between the two groups. Significantly high correlations were found between the age of patients and spouses for both groups of patients, but even stronger correlations were found between sexes for both groups (Table 6.6). This was due to the fact that husbands in both groups tended to have wives slightly younger (2.5 years) than themselves. This assortment of age between couples was in line with the normal population.

Table 6.6 Within Couple Correlation of Age

(Ps,Ss)	0.78 **
(Pn,Sn)	0.87 **
(Ms,Fs)	0.81 **
(Mn,Fn)	0.91 **

** Significant at .05 level

Details of Marriage

The couples of the depressed group had been together in this relationship significantly longer than the schizophrenic group (Table 6.7). This was partly due to the fact that the schizophrenic group (both patients and spouses), were older than the comparison group at the time of first marriage and this marriage (Table 6.8).

Table 6.7 Length of This Marriage

	SCH Group	DEP Group
MEAN (yrs)	13.12	20.88
SD (yrs)	9.71	10.33

Independent T-Test : -2.75 p=.008

Table 6.8 Mean Age when Married

	Patient		Spouse	
	MEAN	SD	MEAN	SD
Age when first married				
SCH Group	31.00	8.48	32.64	11.54
DEP Group	24.68	7.67	24.68	8.54
Age when married this time				
SCH Group	25.42	6.14	27.04	8.33
DEP Group	21.92	3.37	22.16	5.51

Independent T-Test	Ps v Pn	Ss v Sn
Age when first married	p=.016	p=.018
Age when married this time	p=.008	p=.008

84% of the depressed group were actually married for the first time, compared to 66% of the schizophrenic group. Twice as many of the schizophrenic group were married for the second or third time. The schizophrenic patients experienced the largest number of previous marriages, closely followed by the schizophrenic spouses. These rates being approximately double that of the depressed group. There was one spouse in the schizophrenic group who had reported to have had altogether ten marriages (Table 6.9 and Table 6.10).

Table 6.9 Number of Marriage by Patients and Spouses

	SCH Group		DEP Group	
	Patients	Spouses	Patients	Spouses
1st	15 (60%)	18 (72%)	21 (84%)	21 (84%)
2nd	9 (36%)	4 (16%)	4 (16%)	4 (16%)
3rd	1 (4%)	2 (8%)	0 (0%)	0 (0%)
10th	0 (0%)	1 (4%)	0 (0%)	0 (0%)
Total	25 (100%)	25 (100%)	25 (100%)	25 (100%)

Table 6.10 Within-Couple Marriage

	SCH Group				DEP Group		
	Spouse				Spouse		
Patient	1st	Not 1st	Total	Patients	1st	Not 1st	Total
1st	13	2	15	1st	18	3	21
Not 1st	5	5	10	Not 1st	3	1	4
Total	18	7	25	Total	21	4	25

The most common pattern is the first marriage of both partners. When analysed by sex, male schizophrenics tended to have had more previous marriages, but there was no tendency for previously married men schizophrenics to choose partners who had also been married before.

Marriage and First Psychiatric Consultation

Eighty eight percent of the depressed patients but only thirty six percent of schizophrenic patients were married before the patients' first psychiatric consultation. Schizophrenic patients were five times more likely than depressed patients to marry after the first psychiatric consultation (Table 6.11).

Table 6.11 Marriage and First Psychiatric Consultation

	SCH Patient	DEP Patient
Married before 1st consultation	9 (36%)	22 (88%)
Married after 1st consultation	16 (64%)	3 (12%)
Total	25 (100%)	25 (100%)

Chi Square = 14.35 , df = 1 p =.00015

Spouses and Psychiatric Illness

Spouses of the schizophrenic group (28%) were three times as likely as the spouses of the depressed group (8%) to declare that they themselves were also psychiatric sufferers (predominantly husbands in the schizophrenic group) (Table 6.12).

Table 6.12 Spouses Self-Admitted as Psychiatric Sufferer

	SCH Group					DEP Group			
	M	F	Total			M	F	Total	
yes	4	2	6	24%	yes	1	1	2	8%
no	8	11	19	76%	no	11	12	23	92%
Total	12	13	25	100%	Total	12	13	25	100%

Fisher's Exact Test 2-tailed on spouses of two groups declaring themselves psychiatric sufferers : p=.2467

Premarital Situations

Education Level

Couples in the schizophrenic group had slightly more years of education than couples in the depressed group. However, these differences were not statistically significant (Table 6.13). About one fourth of the schizophrenic patients did not know their fathers' education, compared to one eighth of the depressed patients. There were no significant differences between the two diagnostic groups in the respect of education of self, father, and mother. Patients of both groups had significantly more years of education than their own parents, and so did the spouses.

Table 6.13 Years of Education

		SCH Group		DEP Group	
		Patient	Spouse	Patient	Spouse
Self	MEAN	12.40	12.36	10.80	11.72
	SD	2.94	3.16	2.68	3.12
	N	25	25	25	25
Father	MEAN	10.11	9.96	9.09	8.87
	SD	3.78	3.06	2.88	2.24
	N	19	24	22	23
Mother	MEAN	10.30	9.92	9.20	9.32
	SD	3.91	2.47	2.27	2.68
	N	20	24	25	22

Overall, assortment of education (a significant positive correlation) was found only within the parents of both patients and spouses. The correlation between self and father's education was just moderate and did not reach significance. The within couple correlation for all patients was just below a significant level (Table 6.14). However, when analysed by diagnostic group, the schizophrenic group couples differed from the depressed group couples in several ways. First, the patient-spouse assortment was found in the depressed group, but not the schizophrenic group. Second, very strong assortment within parents was found in all sub-group except the spouses of the schizophrenic group. Finally, the patients of the schizophrenic group stood out from other sub-groups as having very minimal relationship with their own fathers' education.

Table 6.14 Within Couple Correlation of Years of Education

	self / father	self / mother	father / mother	self / partner
Combined Groups				
N=40 Patients	0.31	0.17	0.91 **	0.39
N=45 Spouses	0.29	0.26	0.64 **	-0.16
SCH Group				
N=18 Patients	0.10	0.02	0.93 **	0.08
N=24 Spouses	0.24	0.13	0.44	-0.11
DEP Group				
N=22 Patients	0.46	0.25	0.88 **	0.62 *
N=21 Spouses	0.34	0.39	0.92 **	-0.29

*Sig. at .01 level ** Sig. at .05 level

Smoking, Drinking and Drug Taking before This Marriage

In general, more smoker-patients had smoker-spouses and more non-smoker patients had non-smoker spouses for both groups. The within-couple agreement reached significant level for the schizophrenic group, but not for the depressed group (Table 6.15).

Table 6. 15 Smoking Before This Marriage by Diagnostic Groups (paired)

SCH Group

	Spouse	
Patient	yes	no
yes	12	4
no	2	7
Total	14	11

Kappa = 0.50
sig. at .05 level

DEP Group

	Spouse	
Patient	yes	no
yes	9	4
no	4	8
Total	13	12

Kappa = 0.36

The spouses of two groups drank similarly, while the depressed patients drank more frequently than the schizophrenic patients. No pattern of agreement was observed between couples for both groups (Table 6.16).

Table 6.16 Drinking Habit Before This Marriage by Diagnostic Groups (paired)

<u>SCH Group</u>

	Spouses				
Patients	never	seldom	always	Total	
never	1	1	0	2	8%
seldom	3	13	4	20	80%
always	1	2	0	3	12%
Total	5	16	4	25	100%
	20%	64%	16%	100%	

/.. to be continued

DEP Group

Patients	Spouses never	seldom	always	Total	
never	1	0	0	1	4%
seldom	2	12	2	16	64%
always	2	5	1	8	32%
Total	5	17	3	25	100%
	20%	68%	12%	100%	

None of the depressed patients had ever taken any illegal drugs whereas 20% of the schizophrenic patients did admit taking illegal drugs, mostly Cannabis (Table 6.17). A spouse in the depressed group had indicated use of illegal drugs compared with two spouses in the schizophrenic group.

Table 6.17 Illegal Drug Taking Before This Marriage by Illness (paired)

SCH Group

Patients	Spouses yes	no	Total	
yes	1	4	5	20%
no	1	19	20	80%
Total	2	23	25	100%
	8%	92%	100%	

DEP Group

Patients	Spouses yes	no	Total	
yes	0	0	0	0%
no	1	24	25	100%
Total	1	24	25	100%
	4%	96%	100%	

Number of Close Friends Before This Marriage

Spouses of the schizophrenic group had significantly fewer close friends than spouses of the depressed group (Table 6.18). Three spouses and three patients of the schizophrenic group allegedly did not have any close friends at all, compared with only one spouse in the depressed group. Men and women in the schizophrenic group had significantly fewer close friends than their counterparts in the other group (Table 6.19).

Table 6.18 Number of Close Friends Before This Marriage by Diagnostic Group

	SCH Group		DEP Group	
	Patient (Ps)	Spouse (Ss)	Patient (Pn)	Spouse (Sn)
MEAN	5.04	6.56	8.36	13.28
SD	4.33	6.48	8.63	12.03
Number of Close Friends				
none	3	3	0	1
1 - 5	15	12	13	6
6 - 10	6	4	8	6
11 - 15	0	4	2	5
16 - 20	1	1	1	4
21 +	0	1	1	3
Total	25	25	25	25

P value of Independent T-Test on Mean Number of Close Friends

Ps v Ss	0.34	n.s.
Pn v Sn	0.10	n.s.
Ps v Pn	0.09	n.s.
Ss v Sn	0.02	**

(** $p < .05$ level)

Table 6. 19 Number of Close Friends Before This Marriage by Sex

	SCH Group		Depressed Group	
	Male (Ms)	Female (Fs)	Male (Mn)	Female (Fn)
MEAN	6.72	4.88	13.20	8.44
SD	6.32	4.50	13.83	5.36
Number of Close Friends				
none	1	5	0	1
1 - 5	15	12	10	9
6 - 10	5	5	8	6
11 - 15	1	3	0	7
16 - 20	2	0	3	2
21 +	1	0	4	0
Total	25	25	25	25

P value of Independent T-Test on Mean Number of Close Friends

Ms v Fs	0.24
Mn v Fn	0.12
Ms v Mn	0.04
Fs v Fn	0.01

Premarital Family Situations

Although the overall difference did not reach statistical significance, more patients of the schizophrenic group (40%) than of the depressed group (28%) did not live with any of their family members before this marriage. The spouses of the depressed group were twice as likely as the spouses of the schizophrenic group to be living with their family before the marriage. (Table 6.20)

Table 6.20 Lived with Family Members Before This Marriage

SCH Group	Patient (Ps)		Spouse (Ss)	
lived with family members	15	60%	14	56%
not lived with family members	10	40%	11	44%
Total	25	100%	25	100%

DEP Group	Patient (Pn)		Spouse (Sn)	
lived with family members	18	72%	20	80%
not lived with family members	7	28%	5	20%
Total	25	100%	25	100%

	Chi Square, df =1	
Ps v Ss	0.00	n.s.
Pn v Sn	0.11	n.s.
Ps v Pn	0.36	n.s.
Ss v Sn	0.30	n.s.

Most patients groups did not have a conflicting relationship with their parents, but for those who did have a conflicting relationship with their parents, depressed patients were twice the number of schizophrenic patients. (Table 6.21 and Table 6.22)

Table 6.21 Relationship with Parents Before This Marriage by Illness

	SCH Group		DEP Group	
	Patient	Spouse	Patient	Spouse
extreme conflict	2	1	3	1
usually in conflict	1	3	3	3
not bad & not good	6	3	4	8
usually in harmony	9	9	13	10
extreme harmony	7	9	2	3
Total	25	25	25	25

Table 6.22 Relationship with Parents Before This Marriage by Illness (paired)

SCH Group (paired) Patient	Spouse yes	Spouse no	Total	
Yes, conflict with parents	1	2	3	12%
no conflict with parents	3	19	22	88%
Total	4	21	25	100%
	16%	84%	100%	

DEP Group (paired) Patient	Spouse yes	Spouse no	Total	
Yes, conflict with parents	2	4	6	24%
no conflict with parents	2	17	19	76%
Total	4	21	25	100%
	16%	84%	100%	

Courtship

Dating Initiatives

For both diagnostic groups, patients were not different from spouses in *who initiated the dating.* Chi Square test of difference did not indicate any statistical significance. (Table 6.23)

Table 6.23 Who Initiated the Dating by Illness

	SCH Group Patient (Ps)	SCH Group Spouse (Ss)	DEP Group Patient (Pn)	DEP Group Spouse (Sn)	Chi Square	
					Ps v Ss	0.08
me	11	13	12	13	Pn v Sn	0.00
my partner	14	12	13	12	Ps v Pn	0.00
Total	25	25	25	25	Ss v Sn	0.08

Rather, it was predominantly men who initiated the dating. (Table 6.24) 80% men of the schizophrenic group and 84% men of the depressed group indicated that it was they who initiated the dating. The Chi Square test of difference showed significance in distribution by sex in both diagnostic groups.

Table 6.24 Who Initiated the Dating by Sex

	SCH Group		DEP Group		Chi Square	
	Male (Ms)	Female (Fs)	Male (Mn)	Female (Fn)		
					Ms v Fs	18.03 **
me	20	4	21	4	Mn v Fn	20.48 **
my partner	5	21	4	21	Ms v Mn	0.00
Total	25	25	25	25	Fs v Fn	0.00

** Significant at .05 level

For the schizophrenic group, it was about the same proportion of men (44%) rating their wives "hard to get" as to the proportion of women (40%) considering themselves as "hard to get" (Table 6.25). This was also true for the depressed group. For both groups, women were about twice as likely to consider themselves hard to get as men did. It could be said that women were more aware of their own "value" than men. On the other hand, men were also twice as likely as women to consider their partners hard to get. It appeared that women were more likely to be "valued" than men.

Table 6.25 Within Couple Tabulation of Whether One was "Hard To Get"

<u>SCH Group (Male only)</u>

		partner			
		yes	no	Total	
self	yes	2	2	4	16%
	no	9	12	21	84%
	Total	11	14	25	100%
		44%	56%	100%	

/.. to be continued

SCH Group (Female only)

		partner yes	no	Total	
self	yes	3	7	10	40%
	no	2	13	15	60%
	Total	5	20	25	100%
		44%	56%	100%	

DEP Group (Male only)

		partner yes	no	Total	
self	yes	3	2	5	20%
	no	8	12	20	80%
	Total	11	14	25	100%
		44%	56%	100%	

DEP Group (Female only)

		partner yes	no	Total	
self	yes	2	8	10	40%
	no	3	12	15	60%
	Total	5	20	25	100%
		20%	80%	100%	

note : statistical test of independence not carried out because 50% of the cell frequencies were below 5.

About half of the couples of both groups regarded both of them "hard to get" in the courtship. About one third of men considered their wives "hard to get" but not themselves whereas about one third of women considered themselves "hard to get" only, but not their husband. There was one women who considered her husband "hard to get" and herself "easy to get". The pattern was the same for both diagnostic groups (Table 6.26).

Table 6.26 Whether Self and Partner were "Hard to Get"

	SCH Group				DEP Group			
	Male (Ms)		Female (Fs)		Male (Mn)		Female (Fn)	
easy either	2	8%	3	12%	3	12%	2	8%
self hard only	2	8%	7	28%	2	8%	8	32%
partner hard only	9	36%	2	8%	8	32%	3	12%
hard both	12	48%	13	52%	12	48%	12	48%
Total	25	100%	25	100%	25	100%	25	100%

Meeting Place

52% of the couples in the depressed group but only 16% in the schizophrenic group came to know their partners through friends and relatives (Table 6.27). Since it was mentioned before that couples of the schizophrenic group had significantly fewer close friends before this marriage than the depressed group, it was clear that friends and relatives were not a main source of potential mates for the schizophrenic group subjects. On the other hand, none of the depressed group but 28% of the schizophrenic group actually came to meet their partner through a hospital or clinic setting. Among the 7 schizophrenic patients who met their partners through hospital or clinic, 5 were married after the 1st psychiatric consultation and 3 of these patients were allegedly without any close friends before this marriage.

Table 6.27 How They First Met

	SCH Patients (Ps)		DEP Patients (Pn)	
friends & relatives	4	16%	13	52%
school or work	3	12%	5	20%
social occasions	7	28%	5	20%
hospital or clinic	7	28%	0	0%
others	4	16%	2	8%
Total	25	100%	25	100%

Parental Satisfaction with Social Lives

According to the subjects' self-report, significantly more parents of the schizophrenic group patients than of the depressed group were satisfied with their children's dating (Table 6.28). Parents of schizophrenic patients were more pleased to see them going out with someone. The frequency distribution was more alike between the spouses of two groups than between patients of two groups.

Table 6.28 Parents' Satisfaction with Your Going Out with Him / Her

	SCH Group				DEP Group			
	Patient (Ps)		Spouse (Ss)		Patient (Pn)		Spouse (Sn)	
not at all	1	4%	6	27%	8	35%	6	24%
a little	4	17%	1	5%	2	9%	2	8%
somewhat	4	17%	5	23%	3	13%	3	12%
quite a lot	5	21%	3	14%	5	22%	7	28%
a great deal	10	42%	7	32%	5	22%	7	28%
n.a.	4		3		2			
Valid Total	24	100%	22	100%	23	100%	25	100%

	Mann-Whitney U	p-value
Ps v Ss	171	0.1293
Pn v Sn	246.5	0.3833
Ps v Pn	149	0.024
Ss v Sn	266.5	0.8519

Choice By Partner

In Table 6.29, overall 56%-80% of the respondent groups thought they had chosen each other equally. Probably more people went for the it when they were given a "middle" way option, However, on the whole, more couples in the depressed group (82%) said so than couples in the schizophrenic group (64%). Couples in the latter group appeared to have less autonomy in the choice of their partner. For both groups, the spouses were twice as likely as the patients to consider that they themselves made the choice. It looked as if when spouses compared to their patient partners felt more autonomy. When analysed by sex (Table 6.30 and Table 6.31), there were more men in the schizophrenic group (28%) than in the depressed group (8%) thought they have chosen their wives. Yet more than half of their wives disagreed. 5 women thought it was their husbands making the choice, 50% of their husbands in the schizophrenic group and 80% of their husbands in the depressed group did not agree. There were some indications of differential restricted autonomy by severity of illness and ill / not ill status, and the universality female choice even among these couples although most of them claimed to choose each other equally in the beginning.

Table 6.29 Who Chose Whom by Diagnostic Groups and Patient/ Spouse

	SCH Group		DEP Group				
	Patient (Ps)	Spouse (Ss)	Patient (Pn)	Spouse (Sn)	*Chi Square*	df =2	
I more	3	6	1	2	Ps v Ss	1.61	n.s.
she more	4	5	2	4	Pn v Sn	1.22	n.s.
we equally	18	14	22	19	Ps v Pn	2.07	n.s.
Total	25	25	25	25	Ss v Sn	2.87	n.s.

Table 6.30 Who Chose Whom by Illness and Sex

	SCH Group		DEP Group				
	Male (Ms)	Female (Fs)	Male (Mn)	Female (Fn)	*Chi Square*	df =2	
I more	7	2	2	1	Ms v Fs	3.90	n.s.
she more	3	6	1	5	Mn v Fn	3.22	n.s.
we equally	15	17	22	19	Ms v Mn	5.10	n.s.
Total	25	25	25	25	Fs v Fn	0.54	n.s.

Table 6.31 Who Chose Whom by Illness and Sex (paired)

SCH Group (paired)

Male	Female I	he	we	Total	Partner	she disagree	he disagree
I more	0	3	4	7	I	4	0
she more	2	0	1	3	he / she	1	3
we equally	0	3	12	15	we	3	5
Total	2	6	17	25	Total	8	8

DEP Group (paired)

Male	Female I	he	we	Total	Partner	she disagree	he disagree
I more	0	1	1	2	I more	1	1
she more	0	0	1	1	He /she	1	4
we equally	1	4	17	22	we	5	2
Total	1	5	19	25	Total	7	7

Interpersonal Attraction in Courtship

Women in the schizophrenic group were significantly lower in mean score for eyes and face (Mean=3.44, SD=1.12) and build / body shape (Mean=3.08, SD=1.32) than their own husbands. For the depressed group, men had a different taste. They had valued significantly more on the dress (Mean=4.04, SD=0.98) and manner (Mean=4.52, SD=0.59) than their women. When the men in the schizophrenic group were compared with the men in the depressed group, the latter group had a significantly higher mean in *eyes and face.* The same pattern held true for the women in both groups. When the two diagnostic groups were combined to men and women only, it was clear that men treasured significantly physical appearance (more the eyes and face, body shape) and overall attraction of their partners than women did. These results were in agreement with the thesis that men were attracted by women's beauty. However as far as education was concerned, it was interesting to find that women in the two diagnostic groups had slightly different expectations. Women in the schizophrenic group valued slightly more in education of the partners (Mean=3.16, SD=1.49) than their men did (Mean=3.04, SD=1.46) while women in the depressed group had a much lower expectation in the education of the partners(Mean=2.48, SD=1.50). This made the combined group score for women (Mean=2.82, SD=1.52) significantly lower than that of men (Mean=3.14, SD=1.41). (Please refer to Table 6.32 and Table 6.33 for details)

Table 6.32 Mean Scores of Attraction Items

	SCH Group		DEP Group		All Groups	
	M	F	M	F	M	F
	Mean (SD)	Mean (SD)	Mean (SD)	Mean (SD)	Mean (SD)	Mean (SD)
(ATT1) dress / clothing	3.80 (10.88)	3.04 (1.46)	4.04 (0.98)	3.16 (1.11)	3.80 (1.09)	3.10 (1.28)
(ATT2) eyes and face	4.32 (0.79)	3.44 (1.12)	4.60 (0.58)	4.36 (0.81)	4.32 (0.79)	3.90 (1.07)
(ATT3) build / body shape	3.88 (1.17)	3.08 (1.32)	4.12 (0.93)	3.68 (1.28)	4.00 (1.05)	3.38 (1.32)
(ATT4) education	3.04 (1.46)	3.16 (1.49)	3.24 (1.39)	2.48 (1.50)	3.14 (1.41)	2.82 (1.52)
(ATT5) voice	3.76 (1.23)	3.40 (1.35)	3.56 (1.12)	3.72 (1.06)	3.66 (1.17)	3.56 (1.22)
(ATT6) job	2.12 (1.33)	2.16 (1.38)	2.88 (1.45)	2.68 (1.38)	2.50 (1.43)	2.41 (1.36)
(ATT7) manner	4.44 (0.77)	4.24 (0.93)	4.52 (0.59)	3.92 (1.19)	4.48 (0.68)	4.08 (1.07)
(ATT8) overall attractiveness	4.60 (0.58)	4.16 (0.94)	4.56 (0.71)	4.56 (0.58)	4.58 (0.64)	4.36 (0.82)

Table 6.33 Summary of Independent T-Test on Attraction Scores

	Ms v Fs	Mn v Fn	Ms v Mn	Fs v Fn	M v F
(ATT1) dress	n.s.	**	n.s.	n.s.	n.s.
(ATT2) eyes & face	**	n.s.	**	**	**
(ATT3) body shape	**	n.s.	n.s.	n.s.	**
(ATT4) education	n.s.	n.s.	n.s.	n.s.	**
(ATT5) voice	n.s.	n.s.	n.s.	n.s.	n.s.
(ATT6) job	n.s.	n.s.	n.s.	n.s.	n.s.
(ATT7) manner	n.s.	**	n.s.	n.s.	n.s.
(ATT8) overall	n.s.	n.s.	n.s.	n.s.	**

Principal component factor analysis (Table 6.34) yielded three factors on the seven attraction items. Factor one was about Personal Looks which loaded heavily on dress / clothing, and physical attributes like eyes and face, build / body shape. The second factor was about Personal Resources which loaded on one's job and education. The final factor was about Personal Presentation (voice and manner). The three factors accounted for two-third of the variance.

Table 6.34 Eigen Values and Factor Loadings of Attraction Items

Factor	Eigen value	Pct of Var	Cum Pct
1	2.17	31.0	31.0
2	1.32	18.8	49.8
3	1.10	15.7	65.5

Rotated Loadings	Fac.1	Fac.2	Fac.3
dress / clothing	<u>0.56</u>	0.23	0.20
eyes and face	<u>0.79</u>	-0.06	0.25
build / body shape	<u>0.77</u>	0.07	-0.04
education	-0.08	<u>0.86</u>	0.21
voice	0.33	<u>0.74</u>	-0.18
job	0.08	0.26	<u>0.82</u>
manner	0.22	-0.18	<u>0.77</u>

In the dimension of Personal Looks, the schizophrenic group had significantly less interest than the depressed group; men as a whole had a greater interest than women; and patients had a greater concern than spouses. In particular, male depressed patients had a significant interest whereas the women in the schizophrenic group (either patients or spouses) had the least interest in this respect (Please refer to Appendix 1 for analysis of variance of the factor scores).

Considerations For This Marriage

Female schizophrenic patients placed significantly less emphasis on the partners' ability to teach children (MEAN=1.75, SD=1.22), and to provide for a family (MEAN=2.5, S.D=1.88) than the female depressed patients. The female spouses of the schizophrenic patients were found to place significantly less expectation on the partners' ability to provide family finance (MEAN=2.31, SD=1.44) than the female spouses of the depressed patients. (For breakdowns of the mean scores, please refer to Appendix 2). No statistical difference was observed for other areas of considerations (Table 6.35).

Table 6.35 Summary of Test of Difference of Expectations on Partners between Schizophrenic Group and Depressed Group

	Patients		Spouses	
	M	F	M	F
Partner's education	n.s	n.s.	n.s.	n.s.
Partner's family members	n.s.	n.s.	n.s.	n.s.
Partner's ability to teach children	n.s.	**	n.s.	n.s.
Partner's ability to provide finance	n.s.	**	n.s.	**
Partner's willingness to share household chores	n.s.	n.s.	n.s.	n.s.
Partner's ability to get on with my family members	n.s.	n.s.	n.s.	n.s.

** Sig. at .05 level

Major Reasons to Marry

Twenty percent (5 cases) of the female in the schizophrenic group were unable to give any reason for this marriage. The comparison was easier after the categories were collapsed into six areas (Table 6.36) (Please refer to Table 6.37 for exact details). More than half of the respondents of both groups expressed emotional needs (to love or to be loved, to be accepted, wanted to be with her/him etc.) as the major reason. Men in schizophrenic group were twice as likely (22%) as the men in depressed group (11%) to name reasons relating to trust and ease of the relationship. Couples in the depressed group were about one-half (Mn: 3%; Fn: 12%) as likely as couples in schizophrenic group (Ms: 8%; Fs: 20%) to give pragmatic reasons. Couples in the schizophrenic group (Ms, Fs: 12%) were more likely then couples of the depressed group (Mn: 3%, Fn: 0%) to marry because of similarity and compatibility reasons. To marry for the sake of sharing and support, the couples in the schizophrenic group were only half (Ms: 4%; Fs: 5%) as ready as those in depressed group (Mn, Fn: 10%). When regrouped into fewer categories, the Kruskal-Wallis test indicated that the distribution of reasons among the four sub-groups were not the same.

Table 6.36 Major Reasons to Marry (Regrouped and by Sex)

	SCH Group				DEP Group			
	M		F		M		F	
emotional needs	37	54%	35	58%	43	60%	40	58%
similarity/compatibility	8	12%	7	12%	2	3%	0	0%
pragmatic reasons	2	3%	7	12%	6	8%	14	20%
sharing & support	3	4%	3	5%	7	10%	7	10%
trust & ease	15	22%	5	8%	8	11%	7	10%
others	3	4%	3	5%	6	8%	1	1%
	68	100%	60	100%	72	100%	69	100%

Kruskal-Wallis = 10.2117 $p<.01$ one-tailed

Table 6.37 Major Reasons to Marry (Detailed by Sex and Diagnostic Groups)

Reasons	SCH Group				DEP Group			
	M		F		M		F	
I loved him/her	14	21%	19	32%	22	31%	23	33%
He/she accepted me	2	3%	2	3%	0	0%	0	0%
felt lonely/need a companion	8	12%	7	12%	5	7%	4	6%
similar background	1	1%	1	2%	1	1%	0	0%
shared interests	4	6%	4	7%	1	1%	0	0%
compatible	2	3%	0	0%	0	0%	0	0%
attractive	3	4%	2	3%	5	7%	1	1%
easy to get on with	4	6%	0	0%	2	3%	3	4%
good personality / trustworthy	11	16%	5	8%	6	8%	4	6%
pregnant /children	0	0%	4	7%	3	4%	9	13%
away from home	0	0%	2	3%	2	3%	3	4%
parents wanted	0	0%	1	2%	1	1%	0	0%
economic security	2	3%	1	2%	1	1%	2	3%
religion	1	1%	2	3%	0	0%	0	0%
sharing & support	3	4%	3	5%	7	10%	7	10%
Other emotional reasons	13	19%	7	12%	16	22%	13	19%
Total	68	100%	60	100%	72	100%	69	100%

The overall pattern was similar when analysed by patient-spouse (Table 6.38 and Table 6.39). It was clear that the schizophrenic patients (10%) and their spouses (13%) reported reasons of similarity and compatibility more frequently than their counterparts (3%, 0%). On the other hand, the schizophrenic patients were the lowest (3%) among all groups to give pragmatic reasons for the current marriage, but resorted to reasons of trust and ease (18%), three time that of the depressed patients'. This was why the Kruskal-Wallis test of distribution indicated differences among the four sub-groups.

Table 6.38 Major Reasons to Marry (Regrouped and by Patient Status)

	SCH Group				DEP Group			
	Patient		Spouse		Patient		Spouse	
emotional needs	39	57%	33	55%	46	65%	37	53%
similarity/ compatibility	7	10%	8	13%	2	3%	0	0%
pragmatic reasons	2	3%	7	12%	7	10%	13	19%
sharing & support	4	6%	2	3%	10	14%	4	6%
trust & ease	12	18%	8	13%	4	6%	11	16%
others	4	6%	2	3%	2	3%	5	7%
	68	100%	60	100%	71	100%	70	100%

Kruskal-Wallis = 9.1317 $p<.05$ one-tailed

Table 6.39 Major Reasons to Marry (Detailed by Patient Status)

	SCH Group				DEP Group			
	Patient		Spouse		Patient		Spouse	
I loved him/her	15	22%	18	30%	22	31%	23	33%
he/she accepted me	4	6%	0	0%	0	0%	0	0%
felt lonely /need a companion	8	12%	7	12%	7	10%	2	3%
similar background	1	1%	1	2%	1	1%	0	0%
shared interests	4	6%	4	7%	1	1%	0	0%
compatible	1	1%	1	2%	0	0%	0	0%
attractive	3	4%	2	3%	2	3%	4	.6%
easy to get on with	3	4%	1	2%	2	3%	3	4%
good personality /trustworthy	9	13%	7	12%	2	3%	8	11%
pregnant /children	1	1%	3	5%	4	6%	8	11%
away from home	0	0%	2	3%	2	3%	3	4%
parents wanted	1	1%	0	0%	0	0%	1	1%
economic security	1	1%	2	3%	1	1%	2	3%
religion	1	1%	2	3%	0	0%	0	0%
sharing & support	4	6%	2	3%	10	14%	4	6%
Other emotional reasons	12	18%	8	13%	17	24%	12	17%
Total	68	100%	60	100%	71	100%	70	100%

Current Marriage

Marital Satisfaction Among Different Groups

Within the couples, the patients of the schizophrenic group had a significantly higher mean score of satisfaction than their spouses in doing activities together, feeling close to each other, partner's role as a wife/husband, showing affection and concern, and overall satisfaction. There were no such significant differences in the depressed group (Table 6.40 and Table 6.41). It was evident that schizophrenic patients reported a higher satisfaction in the marital relationship than their spouses did.

Table 6.40 Mean Scores of Current Satisfaction Items

	SCH Group		DEP Group	
	Patient(Ps) Mean (SD)	Spouse(Ss) Mean (SD)	Patient(Pn) Mean (SD)	Spouse(Sn) Mean (SD)
doing activities together	4.00 (1.32)	3.40 (1.50)	3.68 (1.15)	3.40 (1.19)
feeling close to each other	4.28 (1.17)	3.72 (1.43)	4.08 (1.22)	4.12 (1.17)
talking and sharing with each other	4.28 (1.06)	3.88 (1.39)	3.76 (1.27)	3.80 (1.08)
own role as husband / wife	3.40 (1.41)	3.84 (1.11)	3.64 (1.35)	4.16 (0.80)
partner's role as husband / wife	4.48 (0.92)	3.76 (1.20)	4.12 (1.20)	4.24 (0.88)
showing affection and concern	4.360 (1.11)	3.68 (1.41)	3.72 (1.28)	4.24 (0.83)
overall satisfaction	4.60 (0.96)	3.88 (1.30)	3.92 (1.26)	4.32 (0.90)

Table 6.41 Summary of Paired T-Test on Items of Marital Satisfaction

	Ps v Ss	Pn v Sn
doing activities together	**	n.s.
feeling close to each other	**	n.s.
talking and sharing with each other	n.s.	n.s.
own role as husband / wife	n.s.	n.s.
Partner's role as husband /wife	**	n.s.
showing affection and concern	**	n.s.
overall satisfaction	**	n.s.

** Sig. at .05 level

When further broken down by sex and by patient-spouse status, the husbands of the depressed patients (MEAN=4.5, SD=0.80) reported a significantly higher satisfaction with their own role as husbands than both the wives of the schizophrenic patients (MEAN=3.75, SD=0.87) and the wives of the depressed patients (MEAN=3.85, SD=0.69) (Table 6.42 and Table 6.43). As far as the patients were concerned, the male depressed patients reported a significantly higher satisfaction of doing activities together (MEAN=4.15, SD=1.07) than the female depressed patients (MEAN=3.16, SD=1.03).

Table 6.42 Summary of Independent T-Test of Difference of Satisfaction with Current Marriage by Sex and by Patient-Spouse Status

	(a)	(b)	(c)	(d)	(e)	(f)	(g)
Male Patient (SCH v DEP)	n.s	n.s.	n.s.	n.s.	n.s.	n.s.	n.s.
Female Patient (SCH v DEP)	n.s.	n.s.	n.s.	n.s.	n.s.	n.s.	n.s.
Male Spouse (SCH v DEP)	n.s.	n.s.	n.s.	**	n.s.	n.s.	n.s.
Female Spouse (SCH v DEP)	n.s.	n.s.	n.s.	n.s.	n.s.	n.s.	n.s.

keys: (a)= doing activities together; (b)= feeling close to each other; (c)=talking & sharing with each other; (d)= own role as husband/wife; (e)= partner's role as husband/wife; (f)= showing affection and concern; (g)= overall satisfaction

** Sig. at .05 level

Table 6.43 Summary of Independent T-Test of Difference of Satisfaction with Current Marriage by Patient-Spouse Status and by Sex

	(a)	(b)	(c)	(d)	(e)	(f)	(g)
SCH Patient (M v F)	n.s	n.s.	n.s.	n.s.	n.s.	n.s.	n.s.
DEP Patient (M v F)	n.s	n.s.	n.s.	n.s.	n.s.	n.s.	n.s.
Spouse of SCH (M v F)	**	n.s.	n.s.	**	n.s.	n.s.	n.s.
Spouse of DEP (M v F)	n.s.	n.s.	n.s.	n.s.	n.s.	n.s.	n.s.

keys: (a)= doing activities together; (b)= feeling close to each the; (c)=talking & sharing with each other; (d)= own role as husband/wife; (e)= partner's role as husband/wife; (f)= showing affection and concern; (g)= overall satisfaction

** Sig. at .05 level

When the variance of the overall satisfaction was analysed in the dimensions of sex, diagnostic group and patient-spouse status, an interaction effect of group and subject was found. Patients of the schizophrenic group were more satisfied overall than their partners whereas the reverse was true for the depressed group (Appendix 4).

Marital Satisfaction and Current Symptomatology

Among all satisfaction items, the satisfaction with one's own role as a husband or wife was found to have the strongest linear relationship with current symptomatology (-0.24 to -0.31). In general, it was reasonable that the four symptomatology items were negatively correlated with most of the satisfaction items. Among all items of satisfaction, it was interesting to have satisfaction with partner's role only minimally correlated with symptomatology. In other words, the improvement or worsening of symptomatology on oneself did not affect one's evaluation of the partner's role. Only social dysfunction and severe depression ratings had a significant negative linear relation with marital satisfaction. The greater the social dysfunction and severe depression ratings were, the less satisfied one would be with one's own role. It was quite clear and in agreement with other studies on marital satisfaction of ill couples, that current symptomatology had no bearing on overall marital satisfaction (Table 6.44).

Table 6.44 Correlation Coefficients between Marital Satisfaction and Current Symptomatology

N= 100	(a)	(b)	(c)	(d)
doing activities together	0.03	-0.02	0.06	0.09
feeling close to each other	-0.13	-0.21	-0.15	-0.13
talking and sharing with each other	-0.17	-0.21	-0.07	-0.06
own role as husband / wife	-0.24	-0.24	-0.30*	-0.31*
Partner's role as husband / wife	-0.05	-0.10	0.04	-0.01
showing affection and concern	-0.11	-0.14	-0.11	-0.10
overall satisfaction	-0.14	-0.20	-0.05	-0.08

keys: (a)= somatic symptoms; (b)= anxiety & insomnia; (c)= social dysfunction; (d)= severe depression; * Sig. at .01 level

Marital Satisfaction And Personality Dimensions

Most of the correlation coefficients between satisfaction items and personality dimensions were very small. The only exception was that Social Naivety (the re-interpretation of L as social naivety will be explained in the discussion chapter) had a positive and significant linear relationship with one's own role ($r = 0.31$, $p < .01$). The more social naive one was, the more satisfied one would be with one's own role as a husband or wife (Table 6.45).

Table 6.45 Correlation Coefficients between Marital Satisfaction and Personality Traits

N=100	P	E	N	L
doing activities together	0.06	-0.02	0.07	0.08
feeling close to each other	-0.08	-0.03	-0.01	0.15
talking and sharing with each other	0.08	0.06	-0.12	0.12
own role as husband / wife	-0.07	0.13	-0.09	0.31*
Partner's role as husband /wife	0.07	-0.07	-0.01	0.12
showing affection and concern	-0.12	0.05	0.00	0.18
overall satisfaction	0.06	0.08	-0.07	0.15

keys : P = Psychoticism; E = Extroversion; N = Neuroticism; L= Social Naivety; * Sig. at .01 level

Marital Satisfaction and Difference of Age within Couple

Differences in age within the couple did not have any significant linear relationship with the satisfaction items (Table 6.46). When a test of difference was applied to the group where age difference was within five years, and the group more than five years, there were not such significant differences as found in the normal population.

Table 6.46 Correlation Coefficients between Marital Satisfaction and the Difference of Age within Couple (N=50)

doing activities together	0.17
feeling close to each other	0.14
talking and sharing with each other	0.11
own role as husband / wife	0.17
partner's role as husband /wife	-0.00
showing affection and concern	0.15
overall satisfaction	0.13

Hypothetical Choice of Whether One Would Choose The Same Partner Again

The frequency distribution (Table 6.47) illustrated that the majority of both groups gave favourable answer “yes probably” and “yes definitely” to the question whether they would choose the same partner again. 92% of men and 76% of women in the Schizophrenia group indicated a favourable answer compared to 96% of men and 84% of women in the depressed group. Overall, slightly fewer women said so than men. A closer examination indicated that a few women of the Schizophrenia group gave unfavourable answers. This was confirmed with the figures of the analysis of variance on the mean score (Appendix 5). The interaction effect between the diagnostic group and patient-spouse reached significance.

Table 6.47 Frequency Count of Hypothetical Choice of Choosing the Same Partner

	SCH Group				DEP Group			
	Male		Female		Male		Female	
definitely not	0	0%	2	8%	0	0%	0	0%
probably not	1	4%	2	8%	1	4%	2	8%
do not know	1	4%	2	8%	0	0%	2	8%
yes probably	5	20%	4	16%	7	28%	7	28%
yes definitely	18	72%	15	60%	17	68%	14	56%
Total	25	100%	25	100%	25	100%	25	100%

When the answers were collapsed into "favourable" (yes probably, and yes definitely), and "unfavourable" (definitely not, probably not, do not know), the membership could actually be predicted by the satisfaction with one's own role as husband / wife and the satisfaction with the partner's role as husband / wife, with an overall accuracy of eighty four percent (Table 6.48).

Table 6.48 Discriminant Analysis of Favourable and Unfavourable Answers

Correlation between the Discriminant Function and the predicting variables

satisfaction with partner's role as husband / wife	0.93
satisfaction with own role as husband / wife	0.58

Actual Membership		Predicted Membership: unfavourable	favourable
unfavourable	13	10 (76.9%)	3 (23.1%)
favourable	87	13 (13.9%)	74 (85.1%)
Total	100		

84 % cases correctly classified

Further exploration of those being correctly classified discloses that more spouses than the patients are correctly classified. The spouses of the schizophrenic patients are most correctly identified whereas the schizophrenic patients among all sub-groups have the lowest percentage of correct classification (Table 6.49).

Table 6.49 Details of Correct Classification

	Actual Choice			
	favourable	Un-favourable	Total	Within group
SCH Patient	17	1	18	72%
Spouse of SCH Patient	20	3	23	92%
DEP Patients	16	5	21	84%
Spouse of DEP patient	21	1	22	88%
Total	74	10	84	100%
	88%	22%	100%	

7 Building a Social Model

Loglinear modelling has been carried out to ascertain if certain diagnostic variables (patient-spouse status, being psychiatric sufferer or not), had any interaction with social variables (whether first met in medical setting, whether this was the first marriage) and psychometric variables (psychoticism, neuroticism, extroversion, social naivism, GHQ caseness) in determining one's willingness to choose the same partner. There were altogether twenty one viable models involving part or all of each groups of variables. The interaction varied and was beyond statistical modelling at this stage.

From the various results presented in the previous chapter, the couples in the schizophrenic group in general and the schizophrenic patients in particular appeared to be quite different from the comparison group. If these two different groups have their own but different pathway from courtship to marriage and sustaining of marriage, it would be pointless to search for a general model which may suit both groups. On the other hand, since there is evidence that the schizophrenic group are different from the depressed group, it follows that the depressed group (who were selected in sequence with age and sex matched with the schizophrenic patient subjects), may not represent the existing population of the depressives who are still in marriage. For these two reasons, the attempt of finding an acceptable and suitable model would only be justified when it is for the schizophrenic group rather than the depressed group. Nevertheless, it is still worthwhile trying to apply a model that fits the schizophrenic group to the depressed group in order to examine the differences and the possible explanations of such differences.

There are several areas of findings reported in previous chapters which help to start this line of thinking. Firstly, one can only choose a potential mate from the available pool which varies from one person to another. The availability depends on one's social contacts, and also one's ability and capacity to relate to people. In a principal component analysis of a group of social variables, two common factors were found. The first factor is named Social Habits which loaded on three variables that were all before the marriage: drinking habit, smoking habit, and the use of illegal drug (mostly Cannabis). These three variables could indicate to a certain degree, the social exposure and social network. The second factor involved the number of marriages that one had, the length of current marriage, and the number of close friends before marriage, and is termed Relationship Capacity. It involves the general ability to relate intimately to people and to sustain the relationship. The two factors explained half of the total variance of the six variables involved. The details of the factor loadings on these variables are as follows (Table 7.1):

Table 7.1 Rotated Factor Matrix

	Social Habits	Relationship Capacity
drinking habits	-0.73	0.26
smoking habits	0.68	-0.01
the use of illegal drugs	0.60	0.27
length of marriage	0.05	0.87
number of close friends	-0.15	0.60
number of marriage	-0.36	-0.48

Secondly, a striking result was that a considerable number of the schizophrenic patients met their current spouses through the medical setting which represented a new social venue which is made use of by the schizophrenic patients. These three constructs to a large extent reflected the available pools of potential mates and the real opportunities bestowed upon one.

The correlation coefficients between two factor-score variables Social Habits and Relationship Capacity was small (0.12), because of the orthogonal rotation method. The correlation between Met through A Medical Setting and the two factor-variables were similar and were both negative. It simply means that the less active one's social habits, or the less capable one is of an intimate relationship, the more likely that one would meet the partner through the medical setting.

There were no better indicators for one's disadvantaged position in mate selection than one's age at the time of current marriage. The more disadvantaged persons were considered less likely to be able to marry at an earlier age. It was assumed that most people are driven (by whatever forces) to form intimate and confiding relationship whenever possible and situations allowed. The norm in our society was not considered to be the enjoyment of being single, and of course, there are those who would, and do, object to this assumption.

The standardised beta coefficient from Social Habits to the dependent variable was the greatest (-0.45), followed by Met through A Medical Setting (0.31) and relationship capacity (-0.23). It was very reasonable that the more active one's social habits were, the younger one's age would be at the time of current marriage. The reason could well be that wider or more active social habits broadened one's social contacts, and subsequently enlarged the available pool of potential mates. On the other hand, people with greater relationship capacity could make the best use of the opportunities, and hence the more likely to marry at a younger age. All three paths, individually and collectively, were tested to be significantly different from the assumption of zero beta. The error term was below the 0.8 level, and this part of path analysis was considered to be adequate.

The general satisfaction factor was reported in the previous chapter and is included here. It is understood that marital satisfaction was determined by various dynamic factors like communication, financial situation, and role fulfillment. Although there had been reports that the larger difference of age between the couple correlated significantly and positively with marital satisfaction, the results of this study do not support it. Interestingly, age at the time of current marriage regressed significantly and positively on general satisfaction. There are several possible interpretations. Firstly, people who married at a younger age might have higher expectations that were unmet through the relationship. A younger marrying age also signified probably that the first marriage existed through the onset of the illness and the first disruptive experience. Conversely, older marrying age might mean the person had gained more experience from previous marriage, and thus better adjustment skills and more realistic expectations of the partner. For those who did not marry at a younger age, they grew more mature with age, or lowered their expectations both in the search of a partner and after marriage. In either case, they were more likely to be content with one's own marital life.

It is clear that the model in Fig 7.1 better explained the situations of the schizophrenic group, than the model in Fig 7.2 did for the depressed group. With the omission of Met Through Medical Settings in the latter model, the residual error rose significantly (0.22), and the Relationship Capacity did not have a significant effect on one's age at the time of current marriage. This conveys a message that the model is adequate only for the schizophrenic group. It is very probable that the depressed group had pathway very different from the schizophrenic group.

Figure 7.1 A Social Model for Couples of the Schizophrenic Group

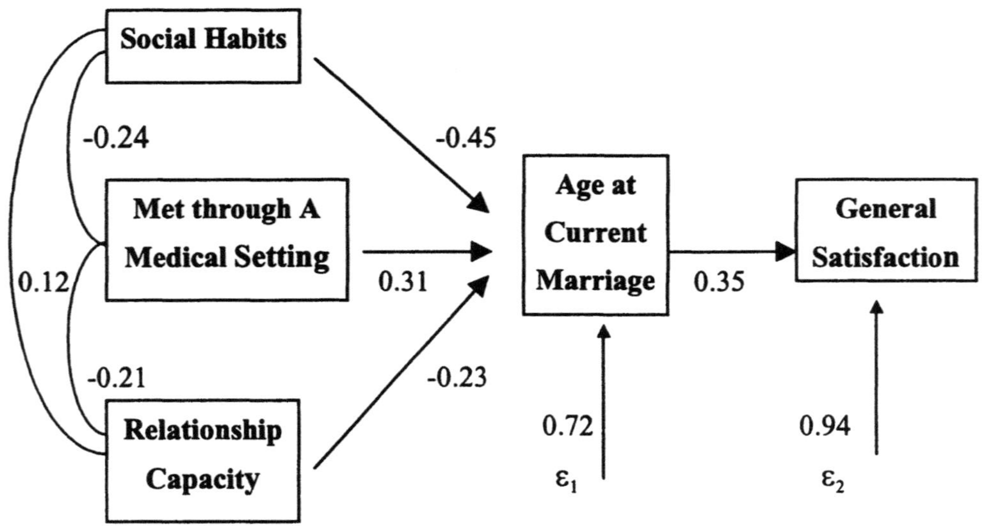

Figure 7.2 A Social Model for Couples of the Depressed Group

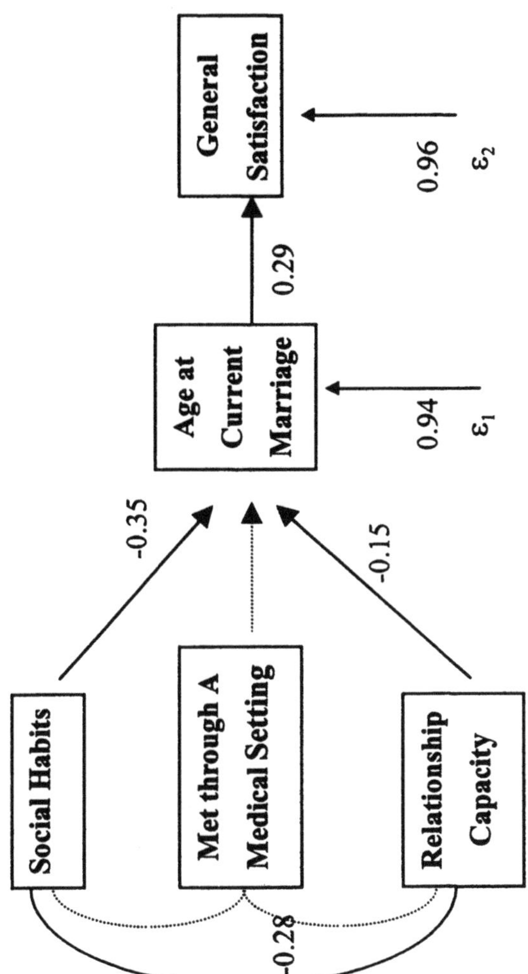

8 Discussion

Sampling and Administering Procedure

Surveys, interviews and tests are all subject to different possible sources of systematic and random error. It is every researcher's hope to reduce or to eliminate systematic errors so that the main variance can be explained by the factors involved, with an acceptable tolerance level of random error. This study identified some possible sources of systematic error prior to its start with regard to the nature of the participants and the research setting. Firstly, it is anticipated that a research study attached to service provision will be more likely to attract people who are in constant contact with the service provision and who may perceive a threat of unfavourable treatment now, or in the future, if they refuse to co-operate in the research study. Such a threat is first reduced considerably by the independence of the researcher who has no part in their treatment or service provision. Second, most patient subjects are ex-patients discharged from the concerned Consultant Psychiatrists within four years; therefore less likelihood of the fear of being rejected of psychiatric services. Third, clear information was provided to the potential participants that the study is not part of treatment, and will not affect in anyway their rights to treatment now or later, and that they are also free to withdraw at any point if they so wish. This should have helped to attract couples who are willing to help in the study, but may also mean that they are more likely to be couples who have adjusted well to their marriage. This may prevent the study from being generalised to those who are married, but are less well adjusted, and to those who are on the edge of break-up. However, judging from the small number of the schizophrenic patients who are with a partner , a sample size of 25 cases actually represents 39% of the cases available to be contacted.

As far as the questionnaire design is concerned, the section of courtship and marriage shall never be intended to become a standard inventory. The question items are exploratory, and should be fine-tuned by subsequent studies to achieve the highest validity. One major weakness of the current design is that the items are too concise and packed into columns. For instance, instead of asking the respondent to rate how impressive their partner was in a number of areas (e.g. hair, dress / clothing, build / body shape etc.) when they first met, it will be more accurate to repeat the same question for each of the areas. The problem here is of course due to the attempt to produce a thin and tidy questionnaire booklet which would not scare away the potential participants.

Undoubtedly, this study has various limitations due to the methodology. The question items on courtship and marriage are far from becoming a standard. The case finding procedures are limited to two major settings of psychiatric rehabilitation, and not all respondents are interviewed. While it is believed that the sample of the schizophrenic group couples represents the schizophrenic group couples, the depressed group couples may not represent the depressed group couples because they are matched only after the schizophrenic group couples are selected. Any finding on the part of the depressed group does not stand on its own to give an accurate profile of the depressed group as a whole. Rather, the depressed group serve only for comparison purpose. Also, extreme cautions must be taken to extend any argument beyond the treated and clinic population, or to make definitive statements on the courtship and marriage of psychiatric patients as a whole.

Psychiatric Illness And Marriage

Disruptive Effect of Psychiatric Illness on Marriage

Although there are no direct explorations of the disruptive effects of psychiatric illness on marriage, some of the results do provide some clues. The schizophrenic patients had more previous marriages, yet had been together for a much shorter period than the depressed patients. It is partly due to the fact that the schizophrenic patients in this study had the current marriage started at an older age, and partly to the fact that some of them had re-established a new confiding relationship after previous break-up. One must remember that the schizophrenic patients in the study represent only a tiny portion who are able to maintain an intimate relationship with lengthy adjustment. The vast majority of single schizophrenics not included in the study could have been either unable to find a partner (Hill et al, 1976) or become single again as a result of marriage break-up. This is confirmed by the comparatively small proportion of schizophrenic patients who were of married or cohabited status, and the much longer period spent in finding schizophrenic patients who still have a partner. Unsurprisingly, the schizophrenic patients experienced the largest number of previous marriages, closely followed by their spouses.

Marriage after First Psychiatric Consultation

One of the striking results is that about two-third of the schizophrenic patients entered the current marriage after their first psychiatric consultation, and this is five times more likely than in the depressed patient group. Given that there were also more schizophrenic patients (40 %) than depressed patients (20%) who had re-married, it appears that the schizophrenic patients are more likely to experience difficulties and problems caused by the illness. However, it is necessary to remember that the majority of the schizophrenic patients were actually married for the first time after the first consultation. That meant the majority of them actually remained single until sometime after the onset of the illness.

Table 8.1 Summary of Percentage of Spouses also Being Ill

	Patients Samples	Community Samples	Mixed Samples
This study	8% [a]		28% [c]
Pond et al (1963)		48% [a]	
Hare & Shaw (1965)		1% [a]	
Hagnell & Kreitman (1974)		15.2% [b]	
Gregory (1959)	6% [a]		
Buck & Ladd (1965)	10.7% [a]		
Kreitman (1964, 1968)	21.3% [b]		
Ovenstone (1973)	30% [a]		
Agulnik (1970)	23%-54% [a] [e]		
Fowler & Tsuang (1975)	38.8% [c] 16.8% [d]		

[a] spouses of neurotic patients only; [b] spouses of all illness; [c] spouses of schizophrenic patients only; [d] spouses of depressive; patients only; [e] partners estimated by scales, not diagnosis or self-report

In this study, more than one-fourth of the spouses (predominantly men) of the schizophrenic patients and 8% of the depressed patients indicated that they were also psychiatric sufferers. For patient samples, neurosis among both couples depended very much on how stringent the diagnostic criteria were. If psychiatric consultation was taken as an acceptable criterion, then the percentage will be between 6% to 10%. This study gave an average of 8%. For community samples in other studies, the variation was even greater depending on the catchment area, and the criteria adopted (Table 8.1).

We cannot be certain what diagnosis would be given to the spouses of our schizophrenic patients. It is probable from the evidence of other studies, that they suffered from various illnesses, different from their partners. In Kreitman's study (1968), only one in nine schizophrenic patients had a partner who was also schizophrenic. It is also interesting to note that Fowler and Tsuang (1975) found an excess rate of schizophrenic patients also having an ill spouse, but none of these ill spouses also suffered from schizophrenia, nor were schizoid-like qualities noted among them.

The schizophrenic patients had a more-than-expected chance of marrying someone who is also ill, (but not belonging to the same diagnostic group). The social aspects of the medical setting may provide an explanation. Usually, medical treatment (in-patient and out-patient) and social rehabilitation are not exclusively for one particular type of sufferer unless special arrangement is made by the medical staff (e.g. psychotherapy group for phobic patients). Patients of various kinds are given new opportunities to make new friendships from within this relatively restricted social environment. The waiting lounge and the drop-in service provide a venue for new friendship.

Thought disorders, social withdrawal, and deficits in social skills are, among other symptoms, the most common and debilitating ones to the social relations of the schizophrenic patients. Very often, they are less responsive, less articulate, and less likely to be interested in other people. These aspects are all essential elements in strengthening existing friendships, and in building new friendships. Lack of volition to relate to people would greatly reduce one's social circle. Even when they meet friends, their deficits in communication skills, and the lack of appropriate affect during interaction, may perhaps produce an unfavourable response from others. For the schizophrenic sufferers, high expressed emotions are more difficult for them to handle and very often they remain in high level of excitement or arousal in face of situation charged with positive or negative expressed emotion (Tarrier et al, 1988; Leff et al, 1989). For the schizophrenic patients who are less able in social contacts, the treatment setting provides an alternative venue where they find less pressure, and communication at a more suitable and "manageable" pace. In this relatively protected environment, the schizophrenic patients are more able to enter into, and sustain, meaningful relationships. Intimate relationships involve essentially a mutually responsive communication which is heavily charged with emotions. By contrast, the cognition, motivation and the ability to relate to others are less affected among depressed patients. The depressed patients already have a wider range of better social connections before entering treatment and they appear to be more able to make new friends from different social occasions. For them, the treatment setting is not such a protected one and they are less likely to enter into courtship and marriage with someone acquainted through the treatment setting.

It will also be important to ask why female schizophrenic patients were more likely than male schizophrenic patients to choose someone who was also ill. One needs to remember that the male-initiative (it is men who approach or start the dating) also applies to the schizophrenic patients. Beauty and looks are assets of women which men valued. The illness had less effect on the resources of women than on the material resources of male schizophrenics (jobs, occupational ability etc.). In several interviews, the husbands of their schizophrenic wives responded in remarkable way when mentioning the looks of their wives at the time they first met. One respondent said, "she's marvellous! Absolutely marvellous!". Another husband burst into a whistle. If courtship and selection of partner is a process of social exchange (Buss & Barnes, 1986; Buss, 1989), the schizophrenic males are doubly handicapped. They do not have the assets that females value and are not motivated to start the exchange process which is mostly male-initiated. It is therefore reasonable to suggest that female schizophrenic patients have a higher chance than male schizophrenic patients do to have a partner, though their illness still puts constraints on their capacity to acquire a non-ill husband.

Social Homogamy

Age

The couples of both the schizophrenic group (r = 0.81) and the depressed group (r = 0.91) were found to be correlated significantly in age within the couple. As expected, the husband-wife correlation of age is above the 0.8 threshold which most anthropometric studies suggested. There is no evidence that the illness altered the general pattern that people tend to choose partners of similar age to them.

Years of Education

Another striking result is the lack of assortment in the area of education level. Although in terms of the years of education received, all patient groups had significantly longer period of education than their own fathers, there was only a moderate linear relationship ($r = 0.31$) between the patients and their fathers. The moderate relationship was due to the very minimal correlation ($r < 0.1$) of the schizophrenic patients. The schizophrenic patients were twice as likely to be unable to recall their fathers' education than the depressed patients, but this cannot explain the low correlation figure of those who did give information on the fathers' education. Obviously, the parental influence which is commonly found in the normal population (Douglas, 1964; Boudon, 1974; Halsey et al, 1980; HMSO, 1989) was not strong in the present study. It is not clear to what extent factors relating to the patients (premorbid intelligence and personality) or factors relating to the educational environment (parental expectation, accessibility to education) are involved. Male schizophrenic patients' year of education had near to zero correlation with their fathers', which contrasted greatly with that between female schizophrenic patients and their own fathers' ($r = 0.64$). It seems that the educational level of the male schizophrenic patients was less influenced by the educational attainment of their fathers. However, there is no evidence that the illness or the disposition of the illness had adversely affected the educational attainment of the patients. It is difficult to decide whether there is a decrease in educational attainment between the subjects and their parents because quite a lot of educational reforms have taken place in 1950s-1970s which would have extended the years of education of this generation in general without necessarily changing their socio-economic status much.

On the other hand, assortment of education within each couple was found among the depressed patients, but not the schizophrenic couples ($r < 0.1$). This suggests that the schizophrenic patients are very different from the normal population in which assortment of education is an important factor in marital choice (Kiser, 1968; Garrison et al, 1968; Johnson et al, 1976; Williams, 1975). As will be discussed later, the partner's education level was not considered of much importance by both patient groups, and when compared, was even less important to the schizophrenic patients than to the depressed patients.

Significant and positive correlation in the years of education received between the parents of all sub-groups were found except the spouses of the schizophrenic group. This particular group of parents were quite contrary to the norm of educational propinquity (Mascie-Taylor, 1987) which might even be more so in last generation where education could mean a rare resource and an important indicator of one's socio-economic status. This leads us to believe that educational achievement was not an important consideration for the parents of the spouses of the schizophrenic patients - a phenomenon found again between the schizophrenic patients and their spouses now.

Social Habits

Assortment by smoking occurs in couples of both diagnostic groups, though only the schizophrenic group reached significant level within the couple. The schizophrenic patients smoked more heavily than their spouses did before the marriage, but the depressed group couples did not differ. Although some studies suggested a relationship between smoking and a specific personality dimension (Spielberger, 1986) and anxiety control (Pritchard & Kay, 1993) in the normal population, there is no information available in this study to ascertain if the same might be true to our patient groups. On the other hand, there is no pattern of agreement or disagreement of drinking within the couple for both groups. The question item in itself was ambivalent and could mean causal or serious drinking, and there is no indication of volume taken. Instead of a real drinking habit, it may simply be an indication of social activity of going to pub.

Illegal drug taking (mostly cannabis) was reported by twenty per cent of schizophrenic patients and eight per cent of their spouses. The proportion is almost the same with the one reported by Fernadez-Pol et al. (1988) among psychiatric sufferers admitted into the hospital (19.8%), but is lower than the one-third estimation of psychostimulant usage (Richard et al, 1985) or the thirty-one per cent incidence rate of overall substance abuse reported by Fischer et al. (1975). The reason for the high proportion in those studies may be accounted for by the presence of more middle class subjects in the samples who were also younger in age (below 25 or below 30) whereas the schizophrenic patients in the study were older, and from a more working-class background. In line with Fernadez-Pol's finding that the schizophrenic patients were less likely to abuse opioids, there is not a single case found among our schizophrenic samples. However, it can be argued that opioid users will have to face more crises in intimate relationships. They have a higher risk of marriage break-up and are more likely not to be included in our samples. While there is very strong evidence of stimulant abuse among younger psychiatric in-patients (Brady et al, 1991; Hovens et al, 1994), the lack of detailed information in the present study on the age when taking cannabis, its frequency and its timing in relation to the onset of illness all make it difficult to ascertain whether such comorbidity really existed when our schizophrenic patients were young. If the depressed patient group in this study are more like the normal population, then the result of the present study is in the same line with two comprehensive reviews (Mueser et al, 1990; Schneier & Siris, 1987) which found that more schizophrenic patients used stimulants and hallucinogens than did the general population.

It is interesting to note that a history of cannabis use in a sample of schizophrenic subjects was associated with significantly lower psychiatric rating on tension and excitement (Mueser et al, 1990). The stimulants act to increase psychological activity and euphoria without the need for a corresponding increase in social activity, and to reduce the tension and excitement that the patients face in the real world. A more recent study by Warner and colleagues (1994) revealed that schizophrenic users of substance (alcohol and cannabis are the two largest groups) cited activity with friends, relief of unpleasant affective states, and boredom as main reasons. In spite of the possible danger of increasing positive symptoms, some schizophrenic users might try to use cannabis in the "best" way to achieve maximal impact on affective symptoms, with minimal increase in positive symptoms.

Social Contacts

It is clear enough that the treatment setting is a social venue for psychiatric patients, and for some of them, it has become a pool of potential mates. This is particularly true for those who had very limited social contacts in their ordinary social network. One may argue that this study only asked about number of close friends before current marriage and not a general indication of total social network, and it may be that people with many friends may not have a few close friends. The analysis of the entire social network of the sample is a separate matter which perhaps deserves another research project. In addition, people who are more motivated (higher extroversion) and have wider social contacts tend to have more close friends. Irrespective of diagnostic group, more patients (80%) than spouses (52%) were classified as low Extroversion group.

Studies of schizophrenia showed that early onset was associated with a higher degree of premorbid behavioural deviance (Offord & Cross, 1969), and deviant men tended to marry schizophrenic women whose schizophrenia began earlier in life. The present study supports this hypothesis by the presence of more female schizophrenic patients of onset at age twenty or before (41%; twice that of male schizophrenic patients and five times that of the female depressed patients). All of these patients were not married for the first time, and they included the three female schizophrenic patients who allegedly had no close friends at all before this marriage. It is very likely that the premorbid deficits in social skills together with the post-morbid deficits played an important part in limiting the available pool and in influencing the choice of a partner whom they met in the treatment setting.

Social Attitudes

It has been demonstrated that within each pair, the spouse did not differ significantly from the patient on the Social Sympathy Scale and the Social Distance Scale. In both groups, the spouses' social sympathy towards mental patients had a positive and significant linear relationship with that of their own partners. Only the couples in the depressed group were not significantly correlated. This similarity is unlikely to be the sole result of choosing a partner whose social attitudes were similar to oneself. Those spouses who had been together with their ill partners were found to be more sympathetic and understanding than those spouses with less than ten years of living together. More lengthy mutual adjustment within the pair did seem to have brought closer the view or reduced the differences over certain attitudes towards mental illness and mental patients. The interaction process involved could be that, through real life experience, the spouses came to know and understand more about mental illness in general and their ill partners in particular. Unnecessary stereotyping could have been avoided through the development of such an understanding. It is also possible that people would try to harmonise psychologically their living experience [with a psychotic patient] with one's cognitive acceptance of mental illness and patients because those who did not sympathise with mental patients would face greater internal incongruence arising from the real experience of having an ill partner. The spouses of the schizophrenic patients seemed to be becoming more sympathetic and keeping less social distance from their ill partners whereas the spouses of the neurotic depressive group were different: they were also as sympathetic as their partners, but some of them preferred to keep a social distance from mental patients and mental illness. Since the two scales measured general attitudes towards mental problems, instead of a particular illness, it is probable that some of spouses of the depressed group did not consider their ill partners as seriously ill as those described in the question items. Congruence may have been achieved through redefining the concept of mental illness, not applying this to their ill partners.

Dating and Making Choice

Initial Attraction and Considerations

It appears to be true for mental patients, regardless of diagnosis, that interpersonal attraction has taken place before the development of an intimate and confiding relationship. The factors derived from initial attraction include Personal Looks, Personal Resources, and Personal Presentation. Men and women loaded differentially on the first two factors. Men placed the overwhelming emphasis on Personal Looks and women placed an emphasis on partners' Personal Resources (i.e. job, education). This is largely in agreement with the differential preference by sex found in the non-clinic population (Buss and Barnes, 1986; Buss, 1989). Although reported as items of attraction, the three factors represent different preferences during different stages of the early contacts. Personal Looks does not require much communication. Personal Presentation includes manner, kindness, and sense of humour that can only be found out during further conversation and contact. For most people, Personal Resources is a matter of concern in a later stage, where more serious evaluation is needed. The three factors represent broadly the stages of initial liking and courtship observed among the non-clinic population (Perper, 1985).

Female Choice

It is predominantly men who started the dating, but it would have been women who made men feel that they were the appropriate target for the men to date – "dateable". For both groups in this study, men were twice as likely as women to consider their own partners hard to get. There was only a tiny proportion of women who considered their husband hard to get and themselves easy to get. It is essentially a matter of male initiative and female choice. This pattern would have been more clearly indicated by the answer to the question "who has chosen whom more" if the subjects had been forced to respond without a middle choice ("we have chosen each other equally"). On the part of men, the majority use of "equal" choice could be interpreted as a socially desirable rationalisation, since they themselves were not the one who made the choice. Nevertheless, the subtlety still can be spotted from the relatively high level of disagreement by the wives to the husbands' claim that they, men made the choice. The rule of the game seems to be: men may feel that they are making the choice but in fact they are not; women are making the choice though they do not admit it!

In spite of the agreement of these general trends in courtship and choice making, the findings of this study do not support the more advanced evolutionist view of social exchange or the so-called human reproductive strategy. One major difference between the present results and other studies is that the female schizophrenic patients and the female spouses in the schizophrenic group did not load on Personal Resources as heavily as the female subjects in the depressed group did. Consistent with this is the significantly low expectation of the husbands of female schizophrenic patients to teach children and to provide family finance. Social exchange theory may be more applicable to and recognisable among the patients of less severe form of mental illness, whose tangible resources remain less affected by the illness.

Personality Traits and Assortative Mating

The Lack of Assortment in Personality Traits

If people choose a partner with similar psychological attributes and if these psychological attributes are relatively stable over time, we will expect to see a high within-couple correlation across those personality dimensions. However, only the neuroticism scores within the couples of the schizophrenic group were positively correlated. On the other hand, if the patients are characterised by certain personality traits and are unlikely to influence their partners, we will expect significant differences within the pairs in the personality traits that concerned. The patients of both groups had a significantly higher N than their own spouses, and for the depressives, the patients had a significantly lower E than their own spouses.

Findings in the previous chapter showed that patient samples in this study were similar to the comparison patient groups provided by the EPQ manual, except that the male schizophrenic patients had a lower mean score in psychoticism than the manual group. There can be a number of reasons for this single difference. First, on the dimensions of psychoticism, different psychotic categories may produce different mean scores. Second, the timing of whether the patient is still an in-patient or discharged when such measurement is taken could have affected the rating. Since about two-third of the patient samples of this study were discharged patients, the mean scores on P was therefore expected to be lower than patients who are still in hospital and under active treatment. Occasionally, a low mean P score was also reported elsewhere (Goh et al, 1982; Kozeny, 1984).

It was clear that overall, the spouses of both the schizophrenic group and the depressed group were not different at all from normal comparison groups of similar age range across the four dimensions of personality, and that individual patient groups were not very different from the comparison patient groups. There is no evidence that the patient subjects had sought a current partner who is similar to them psychologically, nor that a lengthy marital relationship had significantly influenced (diverged or converged) their personality traits.

However, for those spouses of the schizophrenic patients who reported that they were also psychiatric sufferers, they were more like their patient partners than other spouses. They were more neurotic but more introvert than other spouses, and were only different from their patient partners in that they had a higher L mean score. Because of the lack of information on their diagnosis, it is not possible to say whether the schizophrenic patients were more likely to have partner with a particular type of mental illness. In such a small sample, it is very probable that those few spouses are of different diagnostic group.

Reinterpreting L Scale

The interpretation of the Lie scale is far from clear. Since three-quarters of all sample subjects in this study belonged to the high-L group, it deserves a closer examination. In situations like a job interview where the motivation for social desirability is strong, the Lie scale indicates the tendency to dissimulate from normative answers and serves to screen out the high scorers who may distort the responses. The present study is voluntary and without reward. There is little indication that attention from the research worker or the joy of being studied could have motivated them to answer favourably or differently because they knew clearly that there would be no need for any follow-up contact, and that the study has no connection at all with the hospital service they receive. Neither did they know or meet the researcher before the interview. There is no obvious reason that the research process has induced motivation such as dissimulation, except perhaps for a general tendency to wish to please others.

The authors of EPQ (Eysenck and Eysenck, 1975) admitted that the L scale under certain circumstances also measures a different personality dimension - social naivety, a dimension which has seldom been researched. The authors suggested that dissimulation is characterised by a high correlation between N and L (approaching or even exceeding -0.5) whereas small or almost zero correlation indicates little motivation for dissimulation. In the present study, the correlation between N and L is only moderate (-0.27), and dividing the group into high low scores does not make any difference. The removal of the top five percent again does not make much difference. Finally, in spite of a high L mean, other factor means were not abnormally high. This has consequently produced a low PL correlation (-0.11) and a very low EL correlation (-0.009). This suggests that the psychoticism, extroversion, and neuroticism mean scores were not influenced by the L scores. Similarly, L was found to have a low correlation with Social Distance Scale, Social Sympathy Scale, and all GHQ sub-scales. The high mean L appeared not to have influenced the answers to other scales. Sipka et al. (1988) found a similar situation in their study of students attending the military school. The honest and dishonest groups classified by the L scores were not related to behavioural measures of lying and cheating. The L scale shall not therefore be taken automatically as a measure of "flaking good" and this conventional interpretation of L scale as a "lie scale" is unsupported by the present study.

On the other hand, it could be argued, from the content of the items of the scale that the Lie scale also denotes social naivety: a different personality dimension, the nature of which is still not well understood. When the twenty one items of the L scale are looked at, it is not difficult to argue that a considerable number of the questions are concerned with whether one would abstain from or conform to some "socially acceptable deviant" behaviour, like ever cheating, blaming others, breaking promise, pinching things, speaking against others, boasting, taking advantage etc. (i.e. items 4, 8, 13, 16, 24, 35, 39, 48, 51, 59, 63, 69, 89). The other few items are about personal behaviour which may or may not involve other people.

The dissimulation hypothesis assumes that everyone should have committed these socially acceptable deviance, and that high scorers in this dimension are just denying that they ever do these things. Abstaining from "socially acceptable deviance" will appear to be strange or peculiar, judged from the normative view. However it could be the case that these people actually do not do these things, or that they believe they have done them. Assuming that they are not highly religious leaves one with a possible explanation that they are rather socially naive. This could lead them either to respond to these questions positively because they are giving a socially desirable response, or because they actually behave in this way. It is true that a more restricted social network would be less likely to evoke such characteristics (given that they mostly involve interaction with others), but it is also possible that, in same the way, these characteristics may act to reduce the social network, either by putting people off the subject or by the subject being "put off" other people who are socially less naive.

Recent genetic analysis of scale scores both by more conventional factoring (Martin & Jardine, 1986), and the more novel technique of individual item factoring (Heath et al, 1988; 1989a, 1989b) found that the L score had the least genetic influence but the greatest environmental influence (compared to E and N), and that females were more prone to environmental influence. If L is taken as an indication of social naivety, it is possible to suggest that environmental factors like limited social exposure and restricted social network accounted for much variations in this per-sonality dimension. The female schizophrenic patients and the female spouses of schizophrenic patients had the least number of close friends and at the same time were the most naive socially (highest mean L scores) among all sub-groups.

A Social Model of Mate Choice

The findings from the present study do not support the theory of personality needs (complementarity and similarity) (Chapter 2). There is no evidence that the couples had gone through a particular series of stages of relationship, as suggested by sequential theories. The findings are similar to the interpersonal process model in that people have different pathways to an intimate relationship, but unlike the process model, the present study found a restricted social environment played a more important role in influencing one's choice of partner. The sociological theory of propinquity receives more support from the results of the schizophrenic group than from the depressed group, and the social exchange theory appears to be inadequate in explaining the situations of the schizophrenic group. The marriage market theory is probably accurate in describing the difficulties of those who are unable to find a partner, but has not provided satisfactory answers for our married sample. The evolutionist views of reproduction strategy and parental investment (Chapter 3) do not quite describe the treated patient groups and only the social adaptation thesis receives our support.

The model put forth in the previous chapter explains fairly well the general satisfaction variable, for the couples in the schizophrenic group. It may not apply to the couples of the depressed group. The sample size in the present study is not large, but replicating it will be a problem, given the difficulty in acquiring a large number of married schizophrenic subjects. The model is logical and clear in explaining the situational factors that are influencing the consequent success of one's mate choice. What the model has not incorporated is the clinical situation of the patients and partners which may have direct or indirect influence over the "pool-limiting" factors. Research into the mate choice of other diagnostic groups will help to clarify if the same model may or may not apply; and whether different diagnostic groups do have different pathways to their own pool of potential mates. The specific nature of the illness, its relation to the patient's social network and relationship capacity, and the process of rehabilitation may be the major areas that are worth looking into with further research.

Conclusion

The schizophrenic group subjects in the present study appeared to be a very different group from the comparison group. They married at an older age; they had more previous marriages, and fewer close friends. They were more likely to meet through medical setting, but were less able to use the normal venues for creating and sustaining friendship. The saying that "like chooses like" is true in one sense when there were twenty eight per cent of the spouses of the schizophrenic patients also claimed that they were psychiatric patients as well, but they chose others who were quite different from them in education. Neither the compatibility nor complementarity thesis alone can describe adequately the phenomenon.

Clearly the choice of partner is not a random process, nor deterministic matching. The process from acquaintance, to courtship, and to intimacy is very dynamic and is constantly shaped by the psychiatric illness itself, the premorbid and post-morbid social network, and the overall relationship capacity of the parties involved. The illness and premorbid personality may have restricted the social contacts and hence the pool of available mates, but the treatment of the illness opened up new venues of friendship and possibilities for the development of intimate relationships. This is more apparent among schizophrenic patients.

The dating of both groups of patients underwent the similar psychological process of interpersonal attraction and romantic love as in normal subjects, but the expectations on potential mates were more realistic. There is no direct evidence that patients seek partners of similar personality or partners with similar manifestation of symptomatology, but there is a tendency for patients to choose partners of similar life experience and those who would not expect much of them.

The evidence points to the direction of social adaptation of those who suffered from more serious form of psychiatric illness. Though some have experienced disruption of marriage before and have tremendous problems and difficulties in marriage, some others succeeded in creating an intimate relationship and social environment that has more realistic expectations and satisfactions. The results and subsequent discussion are suggestive rather than definitive because of the relatively small sample size, and non-random sampling frame. Future research at the regional or perhaps national level will give a clearer picture.

9 Conclusion

Classical studies of concordance of mental illness among hospital patients or the normal population have left unanswered the question of why and how people with mental illness are more likely to have spouses who are also ill. Some attributed it to initial assortment and hinted at the influence of genetic factors whereas others attributed it to the combination of assortative mating on dispositional factor or marital interaction. This study finds homogamy on certain social variables (non first marriage, social sympathy and social distance towards mental illness), but not on all those personality dimensions which are supposed to be most influenced by genetic factors. On the other hand, the findings do not support either that marital interaction played an important part in determining the personality traits or the symptomatology within the couples.

The process of initial liking and attraction is very much the same as in the normal population. The patients married for various reasons ranging from pragmatic solutions (e.g. pregnancy, wanting children, sharing of resources) to love and life fulfillment. Men are more concerned with looks and physical attractions whereas women are equally concerned with interactional attractions (manner, humor etc.). There is no simple and straightforward picture of exchanging beauty for resources that are advantageous for human reproduction. Female patients seemed to have lowered their expectations on the potential partner and this is more obvious among female schizophrenic patients.

Sex difference still plays a major part in the choice of mate. While it is mostly men who started the initial courtship, it did not follow unanimously that they were the ones who made the choice. Put it more precisely, men believed that they made the choice while women believed that their own consent is more crucial. In this sense, female choice still operates.

As far as the impact of the illness upon the potential to marry and the marriage itself is concerned, the fact that considerable number (64%) of the schizophrenic patients actually married after the first psychiatric consultation and that they are mostly married for the first time and at a later age, reveal the restricted available pool of potential mates that they had. This might be due to the positive and negative symptoms, or the restricted premorbid social environment and / or their deficits in social skills. This study has found it extremely hard to find schizophrenic patients who are still married. Less than ten percent of all the schizophrenic patients are married as indicated by computer record, and out of this small portion, eighty percent have recently separated, divorced or moved. All the evidence points to the impact of the illness in delaying one's courtship and marriage, and the many difficulties that the more severe form of illness like schizophrenia can place in the prospect and the course of marriage.

On the basis of the results, a social model of mate choice is tested and found to explain quite well in statistical and in real terms the situation of the schizophrenic group. Their social network was very much restricted possibly by premorbid personality, and the lack of volition after the onset of the illness. They were less capable to make use of ordinary venues of social contacts for courtship because of their reduced capacity for creating and sustaining relationship.

The present study has not been able to provide any clues as to the breaking up of marriage or whether those who remain single have any particular psychological and social profile, but it has been able to survey those who remain in the intimate relationship. Social adaptation is the key to sustaining relationship. What is needed within the couple is the lowering of expectations, the understanding of one's illness, and greater contentment with one's own role and the role of the partner. One is more likely to find a partner with these characteristics from among those who are also attending psychiatric services. For patients, the medical setting has become a venue as important as other usual social situations, for them to choose and to be chosen. Further study might bring to light the social functions of medical settings and how interpersonal attraction and bonding occurs. Hospital wards, drop-in centres, out-patient clinics and other therapeutic venues might be appropriate places for studying courtship among patients. The pre-sent study suggests that attention may need to be paid to the medical settings (or other residential environment) in its function as a mating pool for disadvantaged patients, such as schizophrenia sufferers. Couturier and Delaunay (1997) observe that hospitals are a meeting point for these seriously ill patients to develop into loving relationships and raise a concern similar to this study, that the psychosocial functions of medical settings have largely been overlooked in the previous studies of assortative mating among patient population.

Amidst the results we found, marital satisfaction is predictable by neuroticism and extroversion, but not psychoticism. However, in none of these three dimensions is the convergence within couples. Success in maintaining the relationship lies not in the compatibility of symptomatology or psychological characteristics within the couples, but by a realistic appraisal of oneself and one's partner. Of course the small sample size of the study does not represent in anyway the many marriage that are facing difficulties and problems. Nevertheless, at least it stands for those who managed to survive the intimate relationship, and it suggests that one does not need to choose someone exactly like them in terms of symptoms, psychoticism, neuroticism, extroversion and social naivety to have a better chance for a more satisfying marriage.

The study has also shed some light on a personality dimension named social naivety which has not been explored much in this context. Most of the existing marriages of the subjects have high level of social naivety, but there is no significant linear relationship within the couples. There are rarely any low-low pairs on social naivety. Female subjects in general, and female schizophrenic patient in particular had significantly higher degree of social naivety. If female choice is one of the golden rules for mate selection, it may well be that this quality among our female subjects has brought a lower demand to the marriage in terms of role expectations. It may also explain why assortment on education level was not found as is so common in the normal population.

Although it is harder for mental patients to get married and survived in an intimate relationship, the couples in this study provide an example of how one can better adapt to the environment by creating a social milieu through marriage that is accepting, understanding, and less demanding. The fittest survive, not the strongest.

Appendices

Appendix 1 Analysis of Variance of the General Factor of Personal Looks

Source of Variation	SS	df	MS	F	Sig
Main Effects	25.46	3	8.49	11.61	0
Group	12.77	1	12.77	17.47	0
Sex	8.63	1	8.67	11.80	0.001
Patient-Spouse	3.60	1	3.60	4.92	0.029
2-way Interactions	3.34	3	1.11	1.52	0.214
Group Sex	0.33	1	0.33	0.46	0.501
Group Patient-Spouse	2.37	1	2.37	3.24	0.075
Sex Patient-Spouse	0.56	1	0.56	0.76	0.385
3-way Interactions	2.95	1	2.95	4.04	0.047
Group Sex Patient-Spouse	2.95	1	2.95	4.04	0.047
Explained	31.75	7	4.54	6.20	0
Residual	67.25	92	0.73		
Total	99	99	1		

Tables of Mean Scores

	Overall	patient	spouse	male	female
SCH group	-0.36	0	-0.72	0.01	-0.72
DEP group	0.36	0.4	0.31	0.59	0.12
patient	0.2			0.41	-0.03
spouse	-0.2			0.18	-0.56
male	0.3				
female	-0.3				

Appendix 2 Mean Scores and Standard Deviations of Considerations for Marriage

		(a)	(b)	(C)	(d)	(e)	(f)
Male Patients							
SCH	MEAN	3.31	2.77	2.39	2.85	3.46	3.46
	SD	1.47	1.48	1.39	1.82	1.33	1.56
DEP	MEAN	1.92	2.54	2.92	2.69	2.92	3.08
	SD	1.12	1.33	1.71	1.60	1.50	1.38
Female Patients							
SCH	MEAN	1.83	2.42	1.75	2.5	3.75	3.42
	SD	1.34	1.62	1.22	1.88	1.60	1.68
DEP	MEAN	2.53	2.58	3.58	4.0	3.17	3.67
	SD	1.43	1.44	1.38	.95	1.75	1.30
Male Spouses							
SCH	MEAN	1.67	2.92	2.71	2.54	3.33	2.58
	SD	1.16	1.68	1.63	1.47	1.44	1.56
DEP	MEAN	2.5	3.0	2.25	2.42	3.0	3.17
	SD	1.62	1.54	1.49	1.51	1.54	1.64
Female Spouses							
SCH	MEAN	2.85	2.69	2.54	2.31	2.92	2.62
	SD	1.35	1.38	1.13	1.44	1.26	1.26
DEP	MEAN	2.15	2.23	3.39	3.85	3.23	3.39
	SD	1.46	1.24	1.45	1.07	1.42	1.50

Keys: (a) partner's education; (b) partner's family members; (c) partner's ability to teach children; (d) partner's ability to provide family finance; (e) partner's willingness to share household chores; (f) partner's ability to get on with one's own family members

Appendix 3 General Factor of Satisfaction before This Marriage

Factor	Eigenvalue	Pct of Var	Cum Pct
1	2.6405	66.0	66.0

Factor Matrix	General Satisfaction
satisfaction with own family life	0.83
satisfaction with own physical health	0.82
satisfaction with own psychological health	0.81
satisfaction with own relationship with relatives	0.80

Analysis of Factor Scores of Satisfaction before This Marriage

Source of Variation	SS	df	MS	F	Sig
Main Effects	6.46	3	2.15	2.21	0.09
Group	4.06	1	4.06	4.17	0.04
Sex	0.09	1	0.09	0.09	0.76
Patient-Spouse	2.28	1	2.28	2.34	0.13
2-way Interactions	2.74	3	0.91	0.94	0.43
Group Sex	0.62	1	0.62	0.64	0.43
Group Patient-Spouse	1.04	1	1.04	1.07	0.30
Sex Patient-Spouse	1.01	1	1.01	1.03	0.31
3-way Interactions	0.25	1	0.25	0.26	0.61
Group Sex Patient-Spouse	0.25	1	0.25	0.26	0.61
Explained	9.45	7	1.35	1.39	0.22
Residual	89.55	92	0.97		
Total	99	99	1		

Appendix 4 Analysis of Variance of Overall Current Satisfaction with Marriage

Source of Variation	SS	df	MS	F	Sig
Main Effects	2.34	3	0.79	0.62	0.61
Group	0.36	1	0.36	0.28	0.60
Sex	1.37	1	1.37	1.07	0.31
Patient-Spouse	0.57	1	0.57	0.44	0.51
2-way Interactions	7.93	3	2.64	2.06	0.11
Group Sex	0.01	1	0.01	0.01	0.92
Group Patient-spouse	7.85	1	7.85	6.12	0.02
Sex Patient-Spouse	0.07	1	0.07	0.06	0.81
3-way Interactions	0.39	1	0.39	0.31	0.58
Group Sex Patient-Spouse	0.39	1	0.39	0.30	0.58
Explained	10.68	7	1.53	1.19	0.32
Residual	118.08	92	1.28	1.31	
Total	128.76	99			

Mean Scores	patient	spouse
Schizophrenic	4.60	3.88
Depressed	3.92	4.32

Appendix 5 Analysis of Variance of Mean Score of Hypothetical Choice of Choosing the Same Partner

Source of Variation	SS	df	MS	F	Sig
	4.91	3	1.64	1.80	0.15
Group	0.25	1	0.25	0.27	0.60
Sex	3.45	1	3.45	3.79	0.06
Patient-Spouse	1.05	1	1.05	1.15	0.29
2-way Interactions	4.70	3	1.57	1.72	0.17
Group Sex	0.17	1	0.17	0.19	0.66
Group Patient-Spouse	4.33	1	4.33	4.76	0.03
Sex Patient-Spouse	0.11	1	0.11	0.12	0.73
3-way Interactions	0.78	1	0.78	0.85	0.36
GRP Sex Patient-Spouse	0.78	1	0.78	0.85	0.36
Explained	10.38	7	1.48	1.63	0.14
Residual	83.81	92	0.91		
Total	94.19	99	0.95		

Mean Scores

	overall	patient	spouse
Schizophrenic	4.36	4.68	4.04
Depressed	4.46	4.36	4.56
male	4.60		
female	4.22		
patient	4.52		
spouse	4.30		

Appendix 6 Courtship and Marriage Questionnaire

Project Information to Participants

This research project is about how you met and came to choose your partner. We want to explore these different patterns of behaviour and compare our findings with those of other studies.

Whether you and your partner agree to take part in the study or not, will not affect your treatment from this hospital / clinic. If you agree to be included in the study, we hope that you and your partner can fill in the questionnaires separately.

You do not need to be interviewed for the study. However, if you have any problems in filling the forms and need some help, our research staff is willing to visit you at home to offer some help. There will be no need for any other contact with you and your partner for the purpose of the study.

All information will be kept completely confidential and your name will not appear anywhere in our documents.

Office use only

			/						

CONSENT FORM

Choice of Partner Study
Department of Psychiatry

I ______________________________________ of (address)
____
____

agree to take part in the choice of partner study that has been explained to me

* in the covering letter / by the staff ____________________
(*delete the one that is inapplicable)

INSTRUCTIONS

There are NO right or wrong answers to each question, and there are NO trick questions throughout the booklet. We would like to know about your own opinions and situation.

Please answer separately on the booklet, one for you and the other for your partner. When you are answering the questions, please do not communicate with your partner.

In the first three pages, please answer every question by writing the numbers in the blanks, putting a tick √ in the box, or ranking in order (1,2,3,4,5) according to the instructions. In the rest of the pages, please underline each of your answers

<u>This part is about your background information</u>

Who is suffering or suffered from the mental illness, you or your partner ?
( ) myself ( ) my partner ( ) both of us

When did you or your partner first receive psychiatric treatment ?
______ (month) 19 ____ (years)

What is your ethnic origin ? _________
( ) British ( ) African ( ) Other European
( ) Indian ( ) Pakistani ( ) Bangladeshi
( ) West Indian ( ) Chinese ( ) Vietnamese
( ) Irish ( ) Others (please specify) ________________

<u>This part is about your family and your own personal details</u>

Name :________________________ Date of Birth: ___/___/ 19__

What is /was your father's occupation ? _______________________

How many years of education did your father receive ? ________ years.

How many years of education did your mother receive ? ________ years.

How many years of education did you receive ? ________ years.

Is this your first marriage / partnership ? Yes____ No____
if no, this is my _______ marriage / partnership.

Date of the start of your first marriage / partnership ___/___/ 19__

Date of the start of this marriage / partnership ___/___/ 19__

When did you first meet your current partner ? in 19____.

Estimate the number of close friends you were in regular contact with before living with your partner ? ______

Did you smoke then ? Yes____ *how many cigarettes a day ? _____
No ____

Did you drink then ?
( ) never
( )occasionally
( ) sometimes
( ) always
( ) daily or almost daily

Did you ever use illegal drugs Yes___ No ___
before living with your partner ? *what drug ? ________________

Did you ever live away from home ?
( ) Yes ( ) No

if yes * for how long ?
( ) less than 3 months
( ) less than 6 months
( ) less than 1 year
( ) less than 2 years
( ) 2 years or more

if yes * under what circumstances ?
( ) in care
( ) in relatives' home
( ) other situation (please specify) ________________________

How would you describe your relationship with your parents ?
( ) extreme conflict ( ) usually in harmony
( ) usually in conflict( ) extreme harmony
( ) not bad and not good

This part is about how you met and dated your current partner.

How did you meet your current partner ?
( ) through friends or relatives
( ) school
( ) work
( ) party or dance
( ) other situations (please specify) ______________________________

With which of your family members did you live with when you met your partner ?
( ) mother or father
( ) both parents
( ) parent and siblings
( ) siblings only
( ) others (please specify) .______________________

Who initiated the dating, you or your partner ?
( ) you ( ) your partner

What did your partner impress you when you two first met ?

Put a number from 1 to 5 beside each of the following
(1= not at all; 2 =a little; 3 =somewhat; 4 =quite a lot; 5 =a great deal)

hair dress / clothing	_____	voice	_____
eyes and face	_____	his / her job	_____
build / body shape	_____	his / her manner	_____
his / her education	_____		

Overall how attractive was your partner ? _____

Name three things about your partner that were most attractive to you.
1. ______________________________
2. ______________________________
3. ______________________________

How far did you think she / he was then :

Put a number from 1 to 5 beside each of the following
(1= strongly disagree; 2 =disagree; 3= uncertain; 4 =agree; 5= strong agree)

physically attractive	_____	educated	_____
sociable	_____	interesting	_____
humorous	_____	gentle	_____
understanding	_____	shared your interest	_____

Were you "hard to get" ?
( ) Yes ( ) No

Was your partner "hard to get" ?
( ) Yes ( ) No

How satisfied were your parents then with your going out with your current partner ?
( ) not at all ( ) a little ( ) somewhat ( ) a lot ( ) very much

<u>This part is about your considerations in making the choice of current partner, and how satisfied you are with a number of situations</u>

Who chose whom ? (tick one box only)
( ) I have chosen my partner more than my partner has chosen me.
( ) my partner has chosen me more than I chose him / her.
( ) we chose each other equally.

When you decided to live with your partner, how important was your consideration about your partner's:

Put a number from 1 to 5 beside each of the following
(1 =not at all; 2 =a little; 3 =somewhat; 4 =quite a lot; 5= very much)

education_____
family members_____
ability to teach children_____
ability to provide family finance_____
willingness to share household chores_____
ability to get on with your family members_____

Before you married / lived together, how satisfied were you with :

Put a number from 1 to 5 beside each of the following
(1 =not at all; 2 =a little; 3 =somewhat; 4 =quite a lot; 5= very much)

your own family life_____
your own physical health_____
your own psychological health_____
your relationship with relatives_____

Give 3 reasons why you decided to marry / live with your current partner.
1. ____
2. ____
3. ____

How satisfied are you now with :

Put a number from 1 to 5 beside each of the following
(1 =not at all; 2 =a little; 3 =somewhat; 4 =quite a lot; 5= very much)

doing activities together_____
feeling close to each other_____
talking and sharing each other_____
your own role as husband / wife_____
your partner's role as wife / husband_____
showing affection and concern to each other_____

Overall how satisfied are you with your married life Now ?_____

If you had the choice now, would you still choose your current partner ?
( ) yes definitely
( ) yes probably
( ) do not know
( ) probably not
( ) definitely not

Bibliography

Abramovitch, R., Finstad, M., Silberfeld, M. (1993), 'Preliminary Report on Informed Consent for Mental Capacity Assessment', *Canadian Journal on Aging*, vol. 12, pp. 373-81.

Abrams, R., Taylor, M.A. (1983), 'The Genetics of Schizophrenia: a reassessment using modern criteria', *American Journal of Psychiatry*, vol. 140, pp. 171-5.

Adler, R. (1995), 'To Tell or Not to Tell: the psychiatrist and child abuse', *Australian and New Zealand Journal of Psychiatry*, vol. 29, pp. 190-98.

Agulnik, P.L. (1970), 'The Spouse of the Phobic Patient', *British Journal of Psychiatry*, vol. 117, pp. 59-67.

Alanen, Y.O., Kinnunen, P. (1975), 'Marriage and the Development of Schizophrenia', *Psychiatry*, vol. 38, pp. 346-65.

Allatt, P., Yeandle, S.M. (1985), *Family Structure and youth Unemployment in an Area of Persistent Decline*, Unpublished Report, University of Durham.

Altman, L.K. (1979), 1 May, The New York Times.

Anderson, W.F. (1992), 'Human Gene Therapy: scientific and ethical considerations', in Chadwick, R.F. (ed.) (revised edition), *Ethics, Reproduction and Genetic Control*, Routlege, London.

Anderson, W.F. (1995), 'Gene Therapy', *Scientific American*, September, pp. 96-9.

Anthony, P. (1989), *The Validity of Informant Reports in Psychiatry*, Ph.D. Thesis, Department of Psychiatry, University of Manchester.

Antill, J.K. (1983), 'Sex Role Complementarity Versus Similarity in Married Couples', *Journal of Personality and Social Psychology*, vol. 45, pp. 145-55.

Appelbaum, P.S. (1997), 'Ethics in Evolution: the incompatibility of clinical and forensic functions', *American Journal of Psychiatry*, vol. 154, pp. 445-6.

Appelbaum, P.S., Grisso, T. (1988), 'Assessing Patients' Capacity to Consent to Treatment', *New England Journal of Medicine*, vol. 319, pp. 1635-8.

Aron, A., Ain, R., Anderson, J.A., Burd, H., Fileman, G., McCallum, R., O'Reilly, E., Rose, A., Stichmann, L., Tamari, Z., Wawro, J., Weinberg, L., Winesauker, J. (1974), 'Relationships with Opposite-Sexed Parents and Mate Choice', *Human Relations*, vol. 27, pp. 17-24.

Artiss, K.L. (1997), Combat Psychiatry: from history to theory, Military Medicine, vol. 162, pp. 605-9.

Bailey, J.M., Gaulin, S., Agyei, Y., Gladue, B.A. (1994), Effects of Gender and Sexual Orientation on Evolutionarily Relevant Aspects of Human Mating Psychology, Journal of Personality and Social Psychology, vol. 66, pp. 1074-80.

Ballinger, C.B. (1975), 'Psychiatric Morbidity and the Menopause : screening of general population sample', *British Journal of Psychiatry*, vol. 131, pp. 83-9.

Ballinger, C.B., Smith, A.H.W., Hobbs, P.R. (1985), 'Factors Associated with Psychiatric Morbidity in Women - a general practice survey', *Acta Psychiatrica Scandinavica*, vol. 71, pp. 272-80.

Banta, T.J., Hetherington, M. (1963), 'Relations between Friends and Fiances', *Journal of Abnormal and Social Psychology*, vol. 66, pp. 401-4.

Barlow, D., Daker, W.G., Band, B. (1997), 'Assortative Sexual Mixing in a Heterosexual Clinic Population - a limiting factor in HIV spread?', AIDS, vol. 11, no.8, pp.1039-44.

Baron, M., Risch, N., Hamburger, R., Mandel, B., Kushner, S. (1987), 'Genetic Linkage between X-chromosome Markers and Bipolar Affective Illness', *Nature*, vol. 326, pp. 289-92.

Barr, C.L., Kennedy, J.L., Pakstis, A.J., Wetterberg, L., Sjogren, B., Bierut, L., Wadelius, C., Wahlstrom, J., Martinsson, T., Guiffra L, Gelernter, J., Hallmayer, J., Moises, H.W., Kurth, J., Cavalli-Sforza, L.L., Kidd, K.K. (1994), 'Progress in a Genome Scan for Linkage in Schizophrenia in a Large Swedish Kindred', *American Journal of Medical Genetics*, vol. 54, pp. 51-8.

Barrett, M. (1980), *Women's Oppression Today*, Verso, London.

Bayer, A.E. (1972), 'College Impact on Marriage', *Journal of Marriage and The Family*, vol. 34, pp. 600-9.

Beauchamp, T.L., Childress, J.F. (2nd ed.), (1982), *Principles of Biomedical Ethics*, Oxford University Press, New York.

Bebbington, P. (1987), 'Marital Status and Depression: a study of English national admission statistics', *Acta Psychiatrica Scandnavica*, vol. 75, pp. 640-50.

Becker, G.S. (1981), *A Treatise on the Family*, Harvard University Press, Boston.

Becker, J. (1963), 'Good Premorbid Schizophrenic Wives and Their Husbands, Family Process', vol. 2, pp. 34-51.

Berger, D.B., Rice, C.E., Sewall, L.G., Lemkan, P.V. (1963), 'Factors Affecting the Adequacy of Patient Community Adjustment Information Obtained from the Community', *Mental Hygiene*, vol. 47, pp. 452-60.

Bernet, W. (1995), 'Running Scared: therapists' excessive concerns about following rules', *Bulletin of the American Academy of Psychiatry and the Law*, vol. 23, pp. 367-74.

Berrettini, W., Ferraro, T., Goldin, L., Weeks, D., Detera-Wadleigh, S., Nurnberger, J., Gershon, E. (1994), 'Chromosome 18 DNA Markers and Manic-Depressive Illness: evidence for a susceptibility gene', *Proceedings of National Academy of Science USA*, vol. 91, pp. 5918-21.

Bertelsen, A., Harvald, B., Hague, M. (1977), 'A Danish Study of Manic-Depressive Disorders', *British Journal of Psychiatry*, vol. 130, pp. 330-51.

Betzig, L.L. (1986), *Despotism and Differential Reproduction: a Darwinian view of history*, Hawthorne, New York.

Bhagat, M. (1976), 'The Spouses of Attempted Suicides : a personality study', *British Journal of Psychiatry*, vol. 128, pp. 44-6.

Billick, S.B., Naylor, P.W., Majeske, M.F., Burgert, I.W. (1996), 'A Clinical Study of Competency in Psychiatric Inpatients', *Bulletin of the American Academy of Psychiatry and the Law*, vol. 24, pp. 505-11.

Billings, P.R., Kohn, M.A., De Cuevas, M., Beckwith, J., Alper, J.S., Natowicz, M.R. (1992), 'Discrimination as a Consequence of Genetic Testing', *American Journal of Human Genetics*, vol. 50, pp. 472-82.

Binder, R.L., McNiel, D.E. (1991), 'Involuntary Patients' Right to Refuse Medication: impact of the Riese decision on a California inpatient unit', *Bulletin of the American Academy of psychiatry and the Law*, vol. 19, pp. 351-7.

Blackwood, D.H.R., He, L., Morris, S. W., et al (1996), 'A Locus for Bipolar Affective Disorder on Chromosome 4p', *Nature Genetics*, vol. 12, pp. 427-30.

Blau, P.M. (1964), *Exchange and Power in Social Life*, Wiley, New York.

Bloch, S., Chodoff, P. (1993), (2nd Edition) *Psychiatric Ethics*, Open University Press, Oxford.

Blood, R.O. Wolfe, D.M. (1960), *Husbands and Wives: the dynamics of married living*, Free Press, New York.

Bolton, C.D. (1961), 'Mate Selection as the Developmental of a Relationship', *Marriage and Family Living*, vol. 23, pp. 234-40.

Borchgrevink, T., Valvik, M. (1983), *En analyse av mor-daster forholdet ag dets betydning for senere parforhold*, Dissertation, University of Oslo.

Botstein, D.R., White, M., Skolnick, M., Davis, R. (1980), 'Construction of a Genetic Linkage Map in Man Using Restriction Fragment Length Polymorphisms', *American Journal of Human Genetics*, vol. 32, pp. 314-31.

Bouchard, T.J., McGue, M. (1990), 'Genetic and Rearing Environmental Influences on Adult Personality: an analysis of adopted twins reared apart', *Journal of Personality*, vol. 58, pp. 263-92.

Boudon, R. (1974), *Education, Opportunity and Social Inequality*, John Wiley & Sons, New York.

Bowlby, J. (1969), *Attachment and Loss*, vol. 1, Institute of Psychoanalysis, Hogarth Press, London.

Brady, K., Casto, S., Lydiard, R.B., Malcolm, R., Arana, G. (1991), 'Substance Abuse in an Inpatient Psychiatric Sample', *American Journal of Drug and Alcohol Abuse*, vol. 17, pp. 389-97.

Brody, B.A., Engelhardt, H.T. (1987), *Bioethics: readings and cases*, Prentice Hall, New Jersey.

Brown, G.W., Harris, T. (1978), *Social Origins of Depression: a study of psychiatric disorder in women*, Tavistock, London.

Buck, C.W., Ladd, K.L. (1965), 'Psychoneurosis in Marital Partners', *British Journal of Psychiatry*, vol. 111, pp. 587-90.

Burgess, E.W., Wallin, P.W. (1953), *Engagement and Marriage*, Lippincott, New York.

Buss, D.M. (1989), 'Sex Differences in Human Mate Preferences: evolutionary hypotheses tested in 37 cultures', *Behavioral and Brain Sciences*, vol. 12, pp. 1-49.

Buss, D.M., Barnes, M. (1986), 'Preferences in Human Mate Selection', *Journal of Personality*, vol. 50, pp. 559-70.

Buss, D.M., Schmitt, D.P. (1993), 'Sexual Strategies Theory: an evolutionary perspective on human mating', *Psychological Review*, vol. 100, pp. 204-32.

Bustamante, C., Gurrieri, S., Smith, S.B. (1993), 'Towards a Molecular Description of Pulsed-Field Gel Electrophoresis', *Trends in Biotechnology*, vol. 11, pp. 23-30.

Cadoret, R.J., Yates, W.R., Troughton, E., Woodworth, G., Stewart, M.A. (1997), 'Genetic-Environmental Interaction in the Genesis of Aggressivity and Conduct Disorders', Archives of General Psychiatry, vol. 52, pp. 916-24.

Callan, V.J. (1983), 'Childlessness and Partner Selection', *Journal of Marriage and The Family*, vol. 45, pp. 181-86.

Campbell, J.B., Reynolds, J.H. (1982), 'Interrelationships of the Eysenck Personality Inventory and the Eysenck Personality Questionnaire', *Educational and Psychological Measurement*, vol. 42, pp. 1066-73.

Carlson, E.A. (1987), 'Eugenics and Basic Genes', *History and Philosophy of Life Sciences*, vol. 3, pp. 57-78.

Carr, D.B., Goate, A., Morris, J.C. (1997), 'Current Concepts in the Pathogenesis of Alzheimer's Disease', *American Journal of Medicine*, vol. 103, Supplement 3A, pp. 3-10.

Cate, R.C., Lloyd, S.A. (1992), *Courtship*, Sage, Newbury Park, California.

Cate, R.M., Huston, T.L., Nesselroade, J.N. (1986), 'Premarital Relationships: Toward the Identification of Alternative pathways to Marriage', *Journal of Social and Clinical Psychology*, vol. 4, pp3-22.

Chan, C.K. (1992), 'Eugenics on the Rise: a report from Singapore', in Chadwick, R.F. (ed.) (revised edition), *Ethics, Reproduction and Genetic Control*, Routlege, London.

Chapman, C.B. (1984), *Physicians, law and Ethics*, New York University Press, New York.

Chasseguet-Smirgel, J. (1964), 'Femine Guilt and Oedipus Complex', in Chasseguet-Smirgel (ed.), *Female Sexuality*, University of Michigan Press, Ann Arbor.

Chodorow, N. (1978), *The Reproduction of Mothering, Psychoanalysis and The Sociology of Gender*, University of California Press, Berkeley.

Collins, F.S. (1995), 'Ahead of Schedule and Under Budget: the Genome Project passes its fifth birthday', *Proceedings of National Academy of Science USA*, vol. 92, pp. 10821-3.

Commins, W.D. (1932), 'The Marriage-Age of Oldest Sons', *Journal of Social Psychology*, vol. 3, pp. 487-9.

Coon, H., Jensen, S., Holik, J., Hoff, M., Myles-Worsely, M., Reimherr, F., Wender, P., Waldo, M., Freeman, R., Leppert, M., Byerley, W. (1994), 'Genomic Scan for Genes Predisposing Schizophrenia', *American Journal of Medical Genetics*, vol. 54, pp. 51-8.

Corder, E.H., Saunder, A.M., Strittmatter, W.J., Schmechel, D.E., Gaskell, P.C., Small, G.W., Roses, A.D., Haines, J.L., Pericak-Vance, M.A. (1993), 'Gene Dose of Apolipoprotein E Type 4 Allele and the Risk of Alzheimer's Disease in Late Onset Families', *Science*, vol. 261, pp. 921-3.

Corser, C.M., Philip, A.E. (1978), 'Emotional Disturbance in Newly Registered General Practice Patients', *British Journal of Psychiatry*, vol. 13, pp. 100-05.

Cournos, F. (1989), 'Involuntary Medication and the Case of Joyce Brown', *Hospital and Community Psychiatry*, vol. 40, pp. 736-40.

Cournos, F. (1993), 'Do Psychiatric Patients Need Greater Protection Than Medical Patients When They Consent to Treatment?', *Psychiatric Quarterly*, vol. 64, pp. 319-29.

Couturier, C., Delaunay, J. (1997), 'Loving Relationships into Psychiatric Institution: freedom or alienation?', (Liens Amoureux En Institution Psychiatrique: Liberte Ou Alienation?), *Annuales Medico Psychologicles*, vol. 155, pp. 217-20.

Craddock, N. (1996), 'Psychiatric Genetics', *British Journal of Psychiatry*, vol. 169, pp. 386-92.

Crow, J.F., Felsenstein, J. (1968), 'The Effect of Assortative Mating on the Genetic Composition of a Population', *Eugenics Quarterly*, vol. 15, No.2, pp. 85-97.

Crow, T.J. (1984), 'A Re-evaluation of the Viral Hypothesis: is psychosis due to retoviral integration at the site of cerebral domance gene?' *British Journal of psychiatry*, vol. 145, pp. 243-53.

Crow, T.J. (1988), 'Aetiology of Psychosis: the way ahead', in Bebbington, P., McGuffin, P. (eds.), *Schizophrenia the major issues*, pp. 127-34, Heinemann, Oxford.

Crow, T.J., (1980), 'Molecular Pathology of Schizophrenia: more than one disease process ?' *British Medical Journal*, vol. 280, pp. 66-8.

Crow, T.J., (1985), 'The Two Syndrome Concept: origins and current states', *Schizophrenia Bulletin*, vol. 11, pp. 471-86.

Crow, T.J., Done, D.J. (1986), 'Age of Onset of Schizophrenia in Siblings: a test of contagion hypothesis', *Psychiatry Research*, vol. 18, pp. 107-17.

Crowe, R.R., Noyes, R., Pauls, D.L., et al. (1983), 'A Family Study of Panic Disorder', *Archives of General Psychiatry*, vol. 40, pp. 1065-069.

Crowe, R.R., Noyes, R., Wilson, A.F., Elston, R.C. et al. (1987), 'A Linkage Study of Panic Disorder', *Archives of General Psychiatry*, vol. 44, pp. 933-7.

Cuber, J.F., Harroff, P.B. (1966), *Sex and the Significant Americans*, Penguin, New York.

Culver, C.M., Gert, B. (1982), *Philosophy in Medicine: conceptual and ethical issues in medicine and psychiatry*, Oxford University Press, New York.

Cummins, W.D. (1932), 'The Marriage-Age of Oldest Sons', *Journal of Social Psychology*, vol. 3, pp. 487-9.

Daly, M., Wilson, M. (1979), *Sex, Evolution and Behavior: Adaptations for Reproduction*, Duxbury, Massachusetts.

Darwin, C. (1958), *The Origin of Species* (6th ed.), New American Library, New York. (Original work published 1859)

Davies, K.E., Pearson, P.L., Harper, P.S., Murray, J.M., O'Brien, T., Sarfrazi, M., Willaimson, R. (1983), 'Linkage Analysis of Two Cloned DNA Sequences Flanking the Duchenne Muscular Dystrophy Locus on the Short Arm of the Human X Chromosome', *Nucleic Acids Research*, vol. 11, pp. 2303-5.

Davison,G.C., Neale, J.M. (1982), *Abnormal Psychology* (3rd ed.), John Wiley, New York.

Dawson, E., Parfitt, E., Roberts, Q., et al. (1995), 'Linkage Studies of Bipolar Disorder in the Region of the Darier's Disease Gene on Chromosome 12q23-24.1. *American Journal of Medical Genetics* (*Neuropsychiatric Genetics*), vol. 60, pp. 94-102.

Dickenson, D. (1997), 'Ethical Issues in Long Term Psychiatric Management', *Journal of Medical Ethics*, vol. 23, pp. 300-4.

DiMaggio, P., Mohr, J. (1985), 'Cultural Capital, Educational Attainment, and Marital Selection', *American Journal of Sociology*, vol. 90, pp. 1231-61.

Douglas, J.W.B. (1964), *The Home and the School*, MacGibbon & Kee, London.

Duck, S.W., Sants, H.K.A. (1983), 'On the Origin of the Specious: Are Personal Relationships Really Interpersonal States?', *Journal of Social and Clinical Psychology*, vol. 1, pp. 27-41.

Dyck, A.J. (1997) , 'Eugenics in Historical and Ethical Perspective', in Kilner, J.F., Pentz, R.D., Young, F.E. (eds.), *Genetic Ethics: do the ends justify the genes?*, Paternoster Press, Michigan.

Dyer, A. (1996), *Ethics and Psychiatry: Towards Professional Definition*, American Psychiatric Association, Washington.

Eckland, B.K. (1968), 'Theories of Mate Selection', *Eugenics Quarterly*, vol. 15, pp. 71-84.

Edwards, J.N. (1969), 'Familial Behavior as Social Exchange', *Journal of Marriage and The Family*, vol. 31, pp. 518-26.

Egeland, J.A., Gerhard, D.S., Pauls, D.L., Sussex, J.N., Kidd, K.K. (1987), 'Bipolar Affective Disorder Linked to DNA Markers on Chromosome 11', *Nature*, vol. 325, pp. 783-7.

Epstein, E., Guttman, R. (1984), 'Mate Selection in Man: Evidence, Theory, and Outcome', *Social Biology*, vol. 31, pp. 243-78.

Essen-Moller, E. (1941), 'Psychiarische Untersuchungen an einer Serie von Zwillingen', *Acta Psychiatrica et Neurologica Scandinavica*, Supplement No.23.

Eysenck, H.J. (1975), 'Personality, Premarital Sexual Permissiveness and Assortative Mating', *Journal of Sex Research*, vol. 10, pp. 47-51.

Eysenck, H.J., Eysenck, S.B.G. (1975), *Manual of the Eysenck Personality Questionnaire (Junior and Adult)*, Hodder & Stoughton, London.

Eysenck, H.J., Eysenck, S.B.G. (1985), *Manual of the Eysenck Personality Scales (EPS Adult)*, Hodder & Stoughton, London.

Farmer, A.E., Jackson, R., McGuffin, P., Storey, P. (1987), 'Cerebral Ventricular Enlargement in Schizophrenia: consistencies and contradictions', *British Journal of Psychiatry*, vol. 150, pp. 324-30.

Femlee, D., Sprecher, S., Bassin, E. (1990), 'The Dissolution of Intimate Relationships: a hazard model', *Social Psychology Quarterly*, vol. 53, pp. 13-30.

Feng, D., Baker, L. (1994), 'Spouse Similarity in Attitudes, Personality, and Psychological Well-Being', Behavior Genetics, vol. 24, pp. 357-64.

Fernadez-Pol, B., Bluestone, H., Mizruchi, M.S. (1988), 'Inner-City Substance Abuse Patterns: a study of psychiatric inpatients', *American Journal of Alcohol Abuse*, vol. 14, pp. 41-50.

Fischer, D.E., Halikas, J.A., Baker, J.W., Smith, J.B. (1975), 'Frequency and Patterns of Drug Abuse in Psychiatric Patients', *Disability and Nerves System*, vol. 36, pp. 550-3.

Fischer, M. (1971), 'Psychosis in the Offspring of Schizophrenic Monozygotic Twins and Their Normal Co-twins', *British Journal of psychiatry*, vol. 118, pp. 43-52.

Fisher, D. (1997), 'Informed Choice: the importance of personal participation in the healing process', in Blackwell, B. (ed.), *Treatment Compliance and the Therapeutic Alliance, Chronic Mental Illness*, pp. 159-69, Harwood Academic Publishers, Singapore.

Fisher, H.E. (1992), *Anatomy of Love, A Natural History of Monogamy, Adultery and Divorce*, Simon and Schuster, London.

Foa, E.B., Foa, U.G. (1980), 'Resource Theory: Interpersonal Behavior as Exchange', in Gergen, K.J.,Greenberg, M.S., Willis, R.H. (eds.), *Social Exchange: Advances in Theory and Research*, pp77-94, Plenum Press, New York.

Fowler, R.C., Tsuang, M.T. (1975), 'Spouses of Schizophrenics: a blind comparative study', *Comprehensive Psychiatry*, vol. 16, pp. 339-42.

Fox, R. (1975), *Encounter with Anthropology*, Peregrine, London.

Freidson, E. (1970), *Professional Dominance: the social structure of medical care*, Atherton Press, New York.

Freimer, N.B., Reus, V.I., Escamilla, M.A., et al. (1996), 'Genetic Mapping Using Haplotype, Association and Linkage Methods Suggests a Locus for Severe Bipolar Disorder (BPI) at 18q22-123', *Nature Genetics*, vol. 12, pp. 436-41.

Freire-Maia, N. (1968), 'Inbreeding Levels in American and Canadian Populations: a comparison with Latin America', *Eugenics Quarterly*, vol. 15, No.1, pp. 22-33.

Freud, S. (1923), *The Ego and The Id*, trans. 1927, reprinted in 1961, in Complete Psychological Works, vol. XIX.

Garrison, G.H., Anderson, V.E., Reed, S.C. (1968), 'Assortative mating' , *Eugenics Quarterly*, vol. 15, pp. 133.

Gershuny, J.I. (1982), 'Household Work Strategies: sexual segregation and Inequality', *Sociological Abstracts*, Supplement, pp. 75.

Gershyny, J.I., Jones, S. (1987), 'The Changing Work / Leisure Balance in Britain 1961-84', *Sociological Review Monograph*, vol. 33, pp. 9-50.

Gert, B., Culver, C.M. (1997), *A Return to Fundamentals*, Oxford University Press, New York.

Gibbs, R.A., Caskey, C.T. (1987), 'Identification and Localization of Mutations at the Lesch-Nyhan Locus by Ribonuclease A Cleavage', *Science*, vol. 236, pp. 303-5.

Gilger, J.W. (1991), 'Differential Assortative mating Found for Academic and Demographic Variables as a Function of Time of Assessment', Behaviour Genetics, vol. 21, pp. 131-50.

Goate, A., Chartier-Harlin, M.C., Mullan, M., Brown, J., Crawford, F., Fidani, L, Haynes, A., Irving, N., James, L., Mant, R., Newton, P., Rooke, K., Roques, P., Talbot, C., Pericak-Vance, M., Roses, A., Williamson, R., Rossor, M., Owen, M., Hardy, J. (1991), 'Segregation of a Missense Mutation in the Amyloid Precursor Protein Gene with Familiar Alzheimer's Disease', *Nature*, vol. 349, pp. 704-7.

Goh, D.S., King, D.W., King, L.A. (1982), 'Psychometric evaluation of the Eysenck Personality Questionnaire', *Educational and Psychological Measurement*, vol. 42, pp. 297-309.

Goldberg, D.P., Hillier, V.F. (1979), 'A Scaled Version of the General Health Questionnaire', *Psychological Medicine*, vol. 9, pp. 139-45.

Goldberg, D.P., Huxley, P. (1980), *Mental Illness in the Community: the pathway to psychiatric care*, Tavistock, London.

Goldman, N., Westoff, C.F., Hammerslough, C. (1984), 'Demography of the Marriage Market in the United States', *Population Index*, vol. 50, pp. 5-25.

Goldsmith, H.H. (1993), 'Nature-Nurture Issues in the Behavioral Genetics Context: overcoming barriers to communication', in Plomin, R., McClearn, G.E. (eds), *Nature Nurture and Psychology*, pp. 325-40.

Gong, Y. (1984), 'Use of the Eysenck Personality Questionnaire in China', *Personality and Individual Differences*, vol. 5, pp. 431-38.

Gottesman, I.I. (1991), *Schizophrenia Genesis: the origins of madness*, Freeman Press, New York.

Gottesman, I.I., Bertelsen, A. (1989a), 'Confirming Unexpressed Genotypes for Schizophrenia: risks in the offspring of Fischer's Danish identical and fraternal discordant twins', *Archives of General Psychiatry*, vol. 46, pp. 867-72.

Gottesman, I.I., Bertelsen, A. (1989b), 'Dual Mating Studies in Psychiatry: offspring of inpatients with examples from reactive (psychogenic) psychoses', *International Review of psychiatry*, vol. 1, pp. 287-96.

Gottesman, I.I., Shields, J. (1972), *Schizophrenia and Genetics: a twin study*, Academic Press, New York.

Gottesman, I.I., Shields, J. (1982), *Schizophrenia: the epigenetic puzzle*, Cambridge University Press, Cambridge.

Greely, H.T. (1992), 'Health Insurance, Employment Discrimination, and the Genetics Revolution', in Kelves, D.J., Hood, L. (eds.), *The Code of Codes: scientific and social issues in the Human Genome Project*, pp. 264-80, Harvard University Press, London.

Greenberg, A.S., Bailey, J.M. (1994), 'The Irrelevance of the Medical Model of Mental Illness to Law and Ethics', *International Journal of Law and Psychiatry*, vol. 17, pp. 153-73.

Gregory, I. (1959), 'Psychiatry, Biological and Social', *Journal of Mental Science*, vol. 105, pp. 457-62.

Grifo, J.A., Giatras, K., Tang, Y.X., Krey, L.C. (1998), 'Successful Outcome with Day 4 embryo Transfer after Preimplantation Diagnosis for Genetically Transmitted Disease', *Human Reproduction*, vol. 13, pp. 1656-9.

Grisso, T., Appelbaum, P.S. (1995), 'MacArthur Treatment Competence Study', *Journal of the American Psychiatric Nurses Association*, vol. 1, pp. 125-7.

Guntrip, H. (1961), *Personality Structure and Human Interaction: The Developing Synthesis of Psychodynamic Theory*, International University Press, New York.

Gusella, J.F., Wexler, N.S., Connerlly, P.M., Naylor, S.L., Anderson, M.A., Tanzi, R.E., Watkins, P.C., Ottina, K. (1983), 'A Polymorphic Marker Genetically Lined to Huntington's Disease', *Nature*, vol. 306, pp. 234-38.

Guttentag, M., Secord, P.F. (1983), *Too Many Women ?* Sage, California.

Hafner, J.R. (1977), 'The Husbands of Agoraphobic Women and Their Influence on Treatment Outcome', *British Journal of Psychiatry*, vol. 131, pp. 289-94.

Hagnell, O., Kreitman, N. (1974), 'Mental Illness in Married Pairs in a Total Population', *British Journal of Psychiatry*, vol. 125, pp. 293-302.

Hallmayer, J., Kennedy, J.L., Wetterberg, L., Sjogren, B., Kidd, K.K., Cavalli-Sforza, L.L. (1992), 'Exclusion of Linkage between the Serotonin 2 Receptor and Schizophrenia in a Large Swedish Kindred', *Archives of General Psychiatry*, vol. 49, pp. 216-9.

Hallmayer, J., Maier, W., Ackenheil, M., Ertl, M.A., Schmidt, S., Minges, J., Lichtmann, D., Wildenauer, D. (1992), 'Evidence against Linkage of Schizophrenia to Chromosome 5q11-q13 Markers in Systematically Ascertained Families', *Biological Psychiatry*, vol. 31, pp. 83-94.

Halsey, A.H., Heath, A., Ridge, J.M. (1980), *Origins and Destinations*, Clarendon Press, Oxford.

Hare, E.H., Shaw, G.K. (1965), 'The Patient's Spouse and Concordance on Neuroticism', *British Journal of Psychiatry*, vol. 111, pp. 102-3.

Harris, H. (1969), 'Enzyme and Protein Polymorphism in Human Populations', *British Medical Bulletin*, vol. 25, pp. 5-13.

Hartman, H. (1981), 'The Family as the Locus of Gender, Class, and Political Struggle', *Signs*, vol. 6, pp. 336-94.

Heath, A.C., Eaves, L.J., Nance, W.E., Corey, L.A. (1987), 'Social Inequality and Assortative Mating: cause or consequence', *Behavior Genetics*, vol. 17, pp. 9-17.

Heath, A.C., Jardine, R., Eaves, L.J., Martin, N.G. (1988), 'The Genetic Structure of Personality I phenotypic factor structure of the EPQ in an Australian sample', *Personality and Individual Differences*, vol. 9, pp. 59-67.

Heath, A.C., Jardine, R., Eaves, L.J., Martin, N.G. (1989a), 'The Genetic Structure of Personality II genetic item analysis of the EPQ', *Personality and Individual Differences*, vol. 10, pp. 615-24.

Heath, A.C., Jardine, R., Martin, N.G. (1989b) 'The Genetic Structure of Personality III multivariate genetic item analysis of the EPQ', *Personality and Individual Differences*, vol. 10, p877-88.

Heston, L.L. (1966), 'Psychiatric Disorders in Foster Home Reared Children of Schizophrenic Mothers', *British Journal of psychiatry*, vol. 112, pp. 819-25.

Hill, C.T., Rubin, Z., Peplau, L. (1976), 'Breakups before Marriage: the end of 103 affairs', *Journal of Social Issues*, vol. 32, pp. 147-68.

Hinde, R.A. (1984), 'Why Do the Sexes Behave Differently in Close Relationship', *Journal of Social and Personal Relationships*, vol. 1, pp. 471-501.

HMSO (1983), *Mental Health Act*.

HMSO (1989), *General Household Survey*, 1986.

Hoffman, B.F., Srinivasan, J. (1992), 'A Study of Competence to Consent to Treatment in a Psychiatric Hospital', *Canadian Journal of Psychiatry*, vol. 37, pp. 179-82.

Hoge, S.K. (1994), 'On being "too crazy" to sign into a mental hospital: the issue of consent to psychiatric hospitalization', *Bulletin of the American Academy of Psychiatry and the Law*, vol. 22, pp. 431-50.

Houlbrooke, R.A. (1984), *The English Family 1450-1700*, Longman, London.

Hovens, J.G., Cantwell, D.P., Kiriakos, R. (1994), 'Psychiatric Comorbidity in Hospitalized Adolescent Substance Abusers', *Journal of American Academy of Child and Adolescent Psychiatry*, vol. 33, pp. 476-483.

Huston, M., Schwartz, P. (1995), 'Lesbian and Gay Male Relationships', in Wood, J.T., Duck, S.W. (eds), Understanding Relationships: off the beaten track, vol. 6, Understanding Relationship Processes, pp. 89-121, Sage, California.

Huston, T.L., Levinger, G. (1978), 'Interpersonal Attraction and Relationships', *Annual Review of Psychology*, vol. 29, pp. 115-56.

Huston, T.L., Surra, C., Fitzgerald, N., Cate, R. (1981), 'From Courtship to Marriage: mate selection as an interpersonal process', in Duck, S., Gilmour, R. (eds.), *Personal Relationships 2: Developing Personal Relationships*, pp. 53-88, Academic Press, London.

Hyman, A., Schillinger, D., Lo, B. (1995), ' Laws Mandating Reporting of Domestic Violence. Do They Promote Patient Well-Being?', *Journal of American Medical Association*, vol. 273, pp. 1781-7.

Jedlicka, D. (1984), 'Indirect Parental Influence on Mate Choice: A Test of Psychoanalytic Theory', *Journal of Marriage and The Family*, vol. 46, pp. 65-70.

Johnson, R.C., Defries, J.C., Wilsin, J.R., McClean, G.E., Vandenberg, S.G., Ashton, G.C., Mi, M.P., Rashad, N.N. (1976), 'Assortative Mating for specific Cognitive Abilities in Two Ethnic Groups', *Human Biology*, vol. 48, pp. 343-52.

Jowell, R., Witherspoon, S. (1985), *British Social Attitudes*, Gower, Aldershot.

Jung, C.G. (1953), *Psychology and Alchemy*, collected works published by Routledge & Kegan Paul, London.

Kallmann, F.J. (1946), 'The Genetic Theory of Schizophrenia: an analysis of 691 schizophrenic twin index families', *Amercian Journal of Psychiatry*, vol. 13, pp. 309-32.

Kalmijn, M. (1991), 'Status Homogamy in the United States', *American Journal of Sociology*, vol. 97, pp. 496-523.

Kaplan, K.H., Price, M. (1989), 'The Clinician's Role in Competency Evaluations', *General Hospital Psychiatry*, vol. 11, pp. 397-403.

Katz, A.M., Hill, R. (1958), 'Residential Propinquity and Marital Selection: A Review of Theory, Method, and Fact', *Journal of Marriage and The Family*, vol. 20, pp. 27-35.

Kelley, H.H., Berscheid, E., Christensen, A., Harvey, J.H., Huston, T.L., Levinger, G., McClintock, E., Peplau, L.A., Peterson, D.R. (1983), *Close Relationships*, Freeman, New York.

Kendler, K.S., Gruenberg, A.M., Tsuang, M.T. (1985), 'Psychiatric Illness in First Degree Relatives of Schizophrenics and Surgical Control Patients', *Archives of General Psychiatry*, vol. 42, pp. 770-9.

Kendler, K.S., Robinette, C.D. (1983), 'Schizophrenia in the National Academy of Sciences - National Research council Twin Registry: a 16-year update', *American Journal of Psychiatry*, vol. 140, pp. 1551-63.

Kenny, J.A., Bounous, R.C. (1961), 'The Psychiatric Patients as his own Historian', *American Journal of Psychiatry*, vol. 118, pp. 341-6.

Kenrick, D.T. (1994), 'Evolutionary Social Psychology: from sexual selection to social cognition', in Zanna, M.P. (ed.), *Advances in Experimental Social Psychology*, vol. 26, pp. 75-122, Academic Press, San Diego.

Kenrick, D.T., Groth, G.E., Trost, M.R., Sadalla, E.K. (1993), Integrating Evolutionary and Social Exchange Perspectives on Relationships: effects of gender, self-appraisal, and involvement level on mate selection', *Journal of Personality and Social Psychology*, vol. 64, pp. 951-69.

Kenrick, D.T., Gutierres, S.E. (1980), 'Contrast Effects and Judgements of Physical Attractiveness: when beauty becomes a social problem', *Journal of Personality and Social Psychology*, vol. 38, pp. 131-40.

Kenrick, D.T., Keefe, R.C. (1989), 'Time to Integrate Sociobiology and Social Psychology', *Behavioral and Brain Sciences*, vol. 12, pp. 24-5.

Kenrick, D.T., Keefe, R.C., Bryan, A., Barr, A., Brown, S. (1995), 'Age Preference and Mate Choice among Homosexuals: a case for modular psychological mechanisms', *Journal of Personality and Social Psychology*, vol. 69, pp. 1166-72.

Kenrick, D.T., Sadalla, E.K., Groth, G., Trost, M.R. (1990), 'Evolution Traits and the Stages of Human Courtship: Qualifying the Parental Investment Model', *Journal of Personality*, vol. 58, pp. 97-117.

Kenrick, D.T., Trost, M.R. (1987), 'A Biosocial Theory of Heterosexual Relationship', in Kelley, K. (ed.), *Women, Men, and Sexuality: theories and research*, pp59-100, State University of New York Press, Albany.

Kenrick, D.T., Trost, M.R. (1989), 'A Reproductive Exchange Model of heterosexual Relationships', in Hendrick, C. (ed.), Close Relationship, *Review of Personality & Social Psychology*, vol. 10, pp. 92-118.

Kenrick, D.T., Trost, M.R. (1993), 'The Evolutionary Perspective', in Beall, A.E., Sternberg, R.J. (eds.), Perspectives on the Psychology of Gender, pp. 148-172, Guilford, New York.

Kenrick, D.T., Trost, M.R. (1997), 'Evolutionary Approaches to Relationships', in Duck, S. (ed.), Handbook of Personal Relationships: theory, research and intervention, (2nd edition), pp. 156-78, Wiley, Chichester.

Kerckhoff, A.C. (1956), 'Notes and Comments on the Meaning of Residential Propinquity as a Factor in Mate Selection', *Social Forces*, vol. 34, pp. 207-13.

Kerckhoff, A.C., Davis, K.E. (1962), 'Value Consensus and Need Complementarity in Mate Selection', *American Sociological Review*, vol. 27, pp. 295-303.

Kerem, B., Rommens, J.M., Buchanan, J.A., Markiewicz, D., Cox, T.K., Chakravarti, A., Buchwald, M., Tsui, L.C. (1989), 'Identification of the Cystic Fibrosis Gene: genetic analysis', *Science*, vol. 245, pp. 1073-80.

Kety, S.S., Rosenthal, D., Wender, P.G., Schulsinger, F. (1968), 'The Types and Prevalence of Mental Illness in the Biological and adoptive Families of Adopted Schizophrenics', *Journal of Psychiatric Research*, vol. 6, pp. 345-62.

Kinsey, A.C., Pomeroy, W.B., Martin, C.E. Gebhard, P.H. (1953), *Sexual Behavior in The Human Female*, Saunders, Philadelphia.

Kirk, C.A., Saunders, M. (1979), 'Psychiatric Illness in a Neurological Outpatient Department in North East England', *Acta Psychiatrica Scandinavica*, vol. 60, pp. 427-37.

Kirkpatrick, C. (1937), 'A Statistical Investigation of the Psychoanalytic Theory of Mate Selection', *Journal of Abnormal Social Psychology*, vol. 32, pp. 427-30.

Kiser, C.V. (1968), 'Assortative Mating by Educational Attainment in Relation to Fertility', *Eugenics Quarterly*, vol. 15, pp. 98-112.

Kjellin, E., Andersson, K., Candefjord, I.L., Palmsteirna, T., Wallsten, T. (1997), 'Ethical Benefits and Costs of Coercion in Short-Term Inpatient Psychiatric Care', *Psychiatric Services*, vol. 48, pp. 1567-70.

Klasper, M.E., Rogers, R., Adams, P.A. (1996), 'Dangerousness and Command Hallucinations: an investigation of psychiatric inpatients', *Bulletin of American Academy of Psychiatry and Law*, vol. 24, pp. 219-24.

Knoppers, B.M., Chadwick, R. (1994), 'The Human Genome Project: under and international ethical microscope', *Science*, vol. 265, pp. 2035-6.

Knuiman, M.W., Divitini, M.L., Bartholomew, H.C., Welborn, T.A. (1996), 'Spouse Correlations in Cardiovascular Risk Factors and the Effect of Marriage Duration', American Journal of Epidemiology, vol. 143, no.1, pp. 48-53.

Kohn, M.L. (1968), 'Social Class and Schizophrenia: a critical review', in Rosenthal, D., Kety, S. (eds.), *The Transmission of Schizophrenia*, Pergamon Press, New York.

Kosa, J., Alpert, J.J., Haggerty, R.J. (1967), 'On the Reliability of Family Health Information', *Social Science and Medicine*, vol. 1, pp. 165-81.

Kozeny, J. (1984), Psychometricke vlastnosti dotazniku EPQ. / 'The psychometric characteristics of the Eysenck Personality Questionnaire', *Ceskoslovenska Psychologie*, vol. 28, pp. 97-115.

Kozeny, J. (1986), 'The GHQ-60 and the EPQ: the content validity', *Activitas Nervosa Superior*, vol. 28, pp. 231-3.

Kreitman, N. (1962), 'Mental Disorder in Married Couples', *Journal of Mental Science*, vol. 108, pp. 438-46.

Kreitman, N. (1964), 'The Patient's Spouse', *British Journal of Psychiatry*, vol. 110, pp. 159-73.

Kreitman, N. (1968), 'Married Couples Admitted to Mental Hospital', *British Journal of Psychiatry*, vol. 114, pp. 699-718.

Kringlen, E. (1967), *Heredity and Environment in the Functional Psychoses*, Heinemann, London.

Laite, J., Halfpenny, P. (1987), 'Employment, Unemployment and the Domestic Division of Labour', in Fryer, D., Ullah, P. (eds.), *Unemployed People*, Open University Press, Milton Keynes.

Lander, E.S. (1996), 'The New Genomics: global views of biology', *Science*, vol. 274, pp. 536-9.

Lander, E.S., Kruglyak, L. (1995), 'Genetic Dissection of Complex Traits: guidelines for interpreting reporting linkage results', *Nature Genetics*, vol. 11, pp. 241-7.

Lander, E.S., Schork, N.J. (1994), 'Genetic Dissection of Complex Traits', Science, vol. 265, pp. 2037-48.

Lasker, G.W. (1968), 'The Occurrence of Identical (Isonymous) Surnames in Various Relationships in Pedigrees: a preliminary analysis of the relation of surname combinations to inbreeding', *American Journal of Human Genetics*, vol. 20, pp. 250-7.

Lasker, G.W. (1985), *Surnames and Genetic Structure*, Cambridge University Press, Cambridge.

Leary, T. (1957), *Interpersonal Diagnosis of Personality*, Ronald, New York.

Ledermann, E.K. (1986), (Revised Edition), *Philosophy and Medicine*, Gower, Hants.

Leff, J., Berkowitz, R., Sharit, N., Strachan, A., Glass, I., Vaughn, C. (1989), 'A Trial of Family Therapy Versus a Relative's Group for Schizophrenia', *British Journal of Psychiatry*, vol. 154, pp. 58-66.

Leigh, G.K., Holman, T.B., Burr, W.R. (1987), 'Some Confusions and Exclusions of the SVR Theory of Dyadic Pairing: a response to Murstein', *Journal of Marriage and the Family*, vol. 49, pp. 933-7.

Lesnik-Oberstein, M., Cohen, L. (1984), 'Cognitive Style, Sensation Seeking and Assortative Mating', *Journal of Personality*, vol. 46, pp. 112-7.

Levine, S., Byrne, K., Wilets, I., Fraser, M., Leal, D., Kato, K. (1994), 'Competency of Geropsychiatric Patients to Consent to Voluntary Hospitalization', American Journal of Geriatric Psychiatry, vol. 2, pp. 300-8.

Levinger, G., Senn, D.J., Jorgensen, B.W. (1970), 'Progress toward Permanence in Courtship: a test of the Kerckhoff-Davis hypotheses', *Sociometry*, vol. 33, pp. 427-43.

Lewis, R.A. Casto, R., Aquilino, W., McGuffin, N. (1978), 'Developmental Transitions in male Sexuality', *The Counseling Psychologist*, vol. 7, pp. 15-9.

Lewis, R.A. (1972), 'A Developmental Framework for the Analysis of Premarital Dyadic Formation', *Family Process*, vol. 11, pp. 17-48.

Lewis, R.A. (1973), 'A Longitudinal Test of a Developmental Framework for Premarital Dyadic Formation', *Journal of Marriage and the Family*, vol. 35, pp. 16-25.

Lidz, T. (1960), 'Family Organization and Personality Structure', in Bell, N.W., Vogel, E.F. (eds.), *A Modern Introduction to The Family*, Free Press, Illinoise.

Lin, M.W., Curtis, D., Williams, N., et al. (1995), 'Suggestive Evidence for Linkage of Schizophrenia to Markers on Chromosome 13q14.1-q32', *Psychiatric Genetics*, vol. 5, pp. 117-26.

Lindley, R. (1988), 'Paternalism and caring', in Fairbairn, G., Fairbairn, S. (eds.) *Ethical Issues in Caring*, Avebury.

Lippert, G.P., Stewart, D.E. (1988), 'The Psychiatrist's Role in Determining Competency to Consent in the General Hospital', *Canadian Journal of Psychiatry*, vol. 33, pp. 250-3.

Lowing, P.A., Mirsky, A.F., Pereira, R. (1983), The Inheritance of Schizophrenic Spectrum Disorders: a reanalysis of the Danish adoptee study data, American Journal of Psychiatry, 140, pp. 1167-71.

Luxenburger, H. (1928), 'Vorlaufiger Bericht uber psychiatrische Serienuntersuchungen an Zwillingen', *Zeitschrift fur die gesamte Neurologie und Psychiatric*, vol. 116, pp. 297-326.

Macciardi, F., Kennedy, J.L., Ruocco, L., Giuffra, L., Carrera, P., Marino, C., Rinaldi, V., Smeraldi, E., Ferrari, M. (1992), 'A genetic Linkage Study of Schizophrenia to Chromosome 5 Markers in a Northern Italian Population, *Biological Psychiatry*, vol. 31, pp. 720-8.

Macciardi, F., Petronis, A., Van Tol, H.H.M., Marino, C., Cavallini, C., Smeradldi, E., Kennedy, J.L. (1994), 'Analysis of the D Sub 4 Dopamine Receptor Gene Variant in an Italian Schizophrenia Kindred', *Archives of General Psychiatry*, vol. 51, pp. 288-93.

Macfarlane, A. (1978), *The Origins of English Individualism*, Blackwell, Oxford.

Machon, R.A., Mednick, S.A., Schulsinger, F. (1983), 'The Interaction of Seasonality, Place of Birth, Genetic Risk and Subsequent Schizophrenia in a High Risk Sample', *British Journal of Psychiatry*, vol. 143, pp. 383-8.

Mainardi, P. (1970), 'The Politics of Housework', in Morgan, R. (ed.), *Sisterhood is Powerful*, pp. 447-54, Vintage, New York.

Manning, S.S., Gaul, C.E. (1997), 'The Ethics of Informed Consent: a critical variable in the self-determination of health and mental health clients', *Social Work in Health Care*, vol. 25, pp. 103-17.

Marshall, D.S. (1971), 'Sexual Behavior on Mangaia', in Marshall, D.S., Suggs, R.C. (eds.), *Human Sexual Behavior: Variations in the Ethnographic Spectrum*, pp. 103-62, Basic Books, New York.

Martin, J., Roberts, C. (1984), *Women and Employment*, Report on the DoE / OPCS Survey, HMSO, London.

Martin, N.G., Jardine, R. (1986), 'Eysenck's Contribution to Behavior Genetics', in Eysenck, H., (ed.) Consensus and Controversy, Falmer Press, London.

Mascie-Taylor, C.G.N. (1987), 'Assortative Mating in a Contemporary British Population', *Annals of Human Biology*, vol. 14, pp. 59-68.

Mascie-Taylor, C.G.N. (1988), 'Assortative Mating for Psychometric Characters', in Mascie-Taylor, C.G.N., Boyce, A.J. (eds.), *Human Mating Patterns*, Society for the Study of Human Biology Symposium 28, Cambridge University Press, Cambridge.

Mascie-Taylor, C.G.N., Vandenberg, S.G. (1988), 'Assortative Mating for IQ and Personality Due to Propinquity and Personal Preference', *Behavior Genetics*, vol. 18, pp. 339-45.

Mathes, E.W., Moore, C.L. (1983), 'Reik's Complementarity Theory of Romantic Love', *Journal of Social Psychology*, vol. 123, pp. 321-7.

Mattinson, J., Ruszczynski, S., Daniell, D., Cohen, N. (1988), *Work, Love and Marriage*, Duckworth, London.

Maule, J. (1998), 'Pulsed-Field Gel Electrophoresis', *Molecular Biotechnology*, vol. 9, pp. 107-26.

Mazur, A., Lamb, T. (1980), 'Testosterone, Status, and Mood in Human Men', *Hormones and Behavior*, vol. 14, pp. 236-46.

McGuffin, P. (1988), 'Genetics of Schizophrenia', in Bebbington, P., McGuffin, P. (eds.), *Schizophrenia: the major issues*, pp. 107-26, Heinemann, Oxford.

McGuffin, P., Reveley, A.M., Holland, A. (1982), 'Identical Triplets: non-identical psychosis?', *British Journal of psychiatry*, vol. 140, pp. 1-6.

McGuffin,P., Farmer, A.E., Gottesman, I.I. (1987), 'Is There Really a Split in Schizophrenia ? The Genetic Evidence', *British Journal of Psychiatry,* vol. 150, pp. 581-92.

McNeill, R.F., Kaij, L. (1978), 'Obstetric Factors in the Development of Schizophrenia: complications in the birth of pre-schizophrenia and in the reproduction of schizophrenic parents', in Wynn, L.C., Chomarsen, R.L., Matthews, S. (eds.) *The Nature of Schizophrenia*, pp. 401-29, Wiley, Chichester.

Mednick, S.A., Schulsinger, F. (1968), 'Some Premorbid Characteristics Related to Breakdown in Children with Schizophrenic Mothers', in Rosenthal, D, Kety, S.S. (eds.), *The Transmission of Schizophrenia*, pp. 267-91, Pergamon, London.

Mehlman, B. (1962), 'Similarity in Friendships', *Journal of Social Psychology*, vol. 57, pp. 195-202.

Merikangas, K.R. (1982), 'Assortative Mating for Psychiatric Disorders and Psychological Traits', *Archives of General Psychiatry*, vol. 39, pp. 1173-80.

Merikangas, K.R., Spiker, D. (1982), 'Assortative Mating among In-Patients with Primary Affective Disorder', *Psychological Medicine*, vol. 12, pp. 753-64.

Messenger, J.C. (1971), 'Sex and Repression in an Irish Folk Community', in Marshall, D.S., Suggs, R.C. (eds.), *Human Sexual Behavior: Variations in the Ethnographic Spectrum*, pp. 3-37, Basic Books, New York.

Michels, R. (1991), 'Psychiatry: where medicine, psychology, and ethics meet', in Browing, D.S., Evison, I.S. (eds.), *Does Psychiatry Need a Public Philosophy*, Nelson-Hall, Chicago.

Miki, Y., Swensen, J., Shattuck-Eidens, D., Futreal, P.A., Harshman, K., Tavtigian, S., Liu, Q, Cochran, C., Bennett, L.M., Ding, W. et al. (1994), 'A Strong Candidate for the Breast and Ovarian Cancer Susceptibility Gene BRCA1', *Science*, vol. 266, pp. 66-71.

Miller, N., Campbell, D.T., Twedt, H., O'Connell, E.J. (1966), 'Similarity, Contrast, and Complementarity in Friendship Choice', *Journal of Personality and Social Psychology*, vol. 3, pp. 3-12.

Moises, H.W., Yang, L., Kristbjarnarson, H., et al. (1995), 'An International Two-Stage Genome-Wide Search for Schizophrenia Susceptibility Genes', *Nature Genetics*, vol. 11, pp. 321-4.

Morris, L. (1985), 'Local Social Network and Domestic Organisation', *Sociological Review*, vol. 33, pp. 327-42.

Morris, L. (1990), *The Workings of the Household*, Polity Press, Cambridge.

Mortensen, D.T. (1988), 'Matching: finding a partner for life or otherwise', *American Journal of Sociology*, vol. 94, Supplement, pp. 215-40.

Mueser, K.T., Yarnold, P.R., Levinson, D.F., Singh, H., Bellack, A.S., Kee, K., Morrison, R.L., Yadalam, K.G. (1990), 'Prevalence of Substance Abuse in Schizophrenia: demographic and clinical correlates', *Schizophrenia Bulletin*, vol. 16, pp. 31-56.

Murray, R.M., Lewis, S. Reveley, A.M. (1985), 'Towards and Aetiological Classification of Schizophrenia', *Lancet*, vol. I, pp. 1023-6.

Murstein, B.I. (1961), 'The Complementary Need Hypothesis in Newlyweds and Middle-Aged Married Couples', *Journal of Abnormal and Social Psychology*, vol. 63, pp. 194-7.

Murstein, B.I. (1970), 'Stimulus-Value-Role: A Theory of Marital Choice', *Journal of Marriage and The Family*, vol. 32, pp. 465-81.

Murstein, B.I. (1976), *Who will Marry Whom ? Theories and Research in Marital Choice*, Springer, New York.

Murstein, B.I. (1987), 'A Clarification and Extension of the SVR Theory of Dyadic Pairing', *Journal of Marriage and the Family*, vol. 49, pp. 929-47.

Naber, D., Kircher, T., Hessel, K. (1996), 'Schizophrenic Patients' Retrospective Attitudes Regarding Involuntary Psychopharmacological Treatment and Restraint', *European Psychiatry*, vol. 11, pp. 7-11.

Negri, F., Melica, A.M., Zuliani, R., Gasperini, M., Macciardi, F., Smeraldi, E. (1981), British Journal of Psychiatry, vol. 138, pp. 236-9.

Nicholson, I.R. (1992), 'A Note on the Generalizability of Assortative Mating Coefficients for Personality', Social Biology, vol. 39, pp.151-7.

Nielsen, J. (1964), 'Mental Disorders in Married Couples (Assortative Mating)', *British Journal of Psychiatry*, vol. 110, pp. 683-97.

National Institute of Health (1998), 'Report of the Joint NIH/DOE Committee to Evaluate the Ethical, Legal, and Social Implications Program of the Human Genome Project', National Human Genome Research Institute.

Normile, D. (1998) 'Medical Ethics: geneticists debate eugenics and China's Infant Health Law', *Science*, 21 August 1998, pp. 1118-9.

Noyes, R., Clarkson, C., Crowe, R.R., Yates, W.R. et al. (1987), 'A Family Study of Generalized Anxiety Disorder', American Journal of Psychiatry, vol. 144, pp. 1019-24.

Oakley, A. (1974), *The Sociology of Home Work*, Robertson, London.

Offord, D.R., Cross, L.A. (1969), 'Behavioral Antecedents of Adult Schizophrenia: a review', *Archives of General Psychiatry*, vol. 21, pp. 267-83.

Ovenston, I.M.K. (1973b), 'The Development of Neurosis in the Wives of Neurotic Men Part II: marital role functions and marital tension', *British Journal of Psychiatry*, vol. 122, pp. 711-7.

Ovenstone, I.M.K. (1973a), 'The Development of Neurosis in the Wives of Neurotic Men: Part I. symptomatology and personality', *British Journal of Psychiatry*, vol. 122, pp. 35-45.

Owen, M.J., McGuffin, P. (1997), 'Genetics and Psychiatry', *British Journal of Psychiatry*, vol. 171, pp. 201-2.

Pahl, R.E. (1971), 'Sociological Portrait: friends and associates', *New Society*, vol. 18, pp. 980-3.

Pahl, R.E. (1984), *Division of Labour*, Basil Blackwell, Oxford.

Pardes, H., Kaufmann, C.A., Pincus, H.A., West, A. (1989), 'Genetics and Psychiatry: past discoveries, current dilemmas, and future directions', *American Journal of Psychiatry*, vol. 146, pp. 435-43.

Parnas, J., Schulsinger, F., Schulsinger, H., Mednick, S.A., Teasdale, T.T. (1982), 'Behavioral Precursors of Schizophrenia Spectrum', *Archives of General Psychiatry*, vol. 39, pp. 658-64.

Parsons, T. (1956), *Family, Socialisation and Interaction Process*, Routledge & Kegan Paul, London.

Patterson, A., P., Weiss, K.D., Noguchi, P.D., Fletcher, J.D. 'In Utero Stem cell Transplantation: clinical and ethical implications', in press.

Paul, D.B. (1994), 'Is Human Genetics Disguised Eugenics?', in Weir, L., Fales, E. (eds), *Genes and Human Self-Knowledge*, pp. 77-8, University of Iowa Press, Iowa.

Peach, C. (1974), 'Homogamy, Propinquity and Segregation: a re-evaluation', *American Sociological Review*, vol. 39, pp. 636-41.

Pekkarinen, P., Bredbacka, P.E., Terwilliger, J., Hovatta, I., Lonnqvist, J., Peltonen, L. (1994), 'Evidence for a Susceptibility Locus for Manic-Depressive Disorder in Xq26', *American Journal of Human Genetic*, vol. 53, pp. 133.

Pekkarinen, P.J.T., Bredbacka, P.E., Loonqvist, J., et al. (1995), 'Evidence of a Predisposing Locus to Bipolar Disorder on Xq24-q27' *Genome Research*, vol. 5, pp. 105-15.

Penrose, L. (1944), 'Mental Illness in Husband and Wife', *Psychiatric Quarterly Supplement*, vol. 18, pp. 161.

Perper, T. (1985), *Sex Signals: the biology of love*, ISI Press, Philadelphia.

Perr, I.N. (1982). 'Refusing treatment – who shall decide', *Bulletin of the American Academy of Psychiatry Law,* vol. 10, pp. 233-47.

Petronis, A., Kennedy, J.L. (1995), 'Unstable Genes, Unstable Mind?', American Journal of Psychiatry, vol. 152. pp. 164-72.

Pitts, F.N., Winokur, G. (1966), 'Affective Disorder, VII: alcoholism and affective disorder', *Journal of Psychiatric Resources,* vol. 4, pp. 37-50.

Pleck, J.H. (1985), *Working Wives, Working Husband*, Sage, Beverly Hills.

Plomin, R. (1990), *Nature and Nurture: an introduction to human behavioral genetics*, Brooks/Cole Publishing, California.

Plomin, R., DeFries, J.C., McClearn, G.E. (1990), *Behavioral Genetics: a primer*, second edition, Freeman, New York.

Polich, M.J. (1982), 'The Validity of Self-Reports in Alcoholism Research', *Addictive Behaviours*, vol. 7, pp. 123-32.

Pollin, W., Stabenau, J.R. (1968), 'Biological, Psychological and Historical Differences in a Series of Monozygotic Twins Discordant for Schizophrenia', in Rosenthal, D., Kety, S.S. (eds.), *The Transmission of Schizophrenia*, Pergamon, Oxford.

Pond, D.A., Ryle, A., Hamilton, M. (1963), 'Marriage and Neurosis in a Working-Class Population', *British Journal of Psychiatry*, vol. 109, pp. 592-8.

Pope, H.G., Jonas, J., Cohen, B.A., Lipinski, J.F. (1983), 'Heritability of Schizophrenia', *American Journal of Psychiatry*, vol. 140, pp. 132-3.

Poythress, N.G., Gascardi, M., Ritterband, L. (1996), 'Capacity to Consent to Voluntary Hospitalization: searching for a satisfactory Zinermon screen', *Bulletin of the American Academy of Psychiatry and the Law*, vol. 24, pp. 439-52.

Pritchard, W.S. Kay, D.L.C. (1993), 'Personality and Smoking Motivation of U.S. Smokers as Measured by The State-Trait Personality Inventory, The Eysenck Personality Questionnaire, and Spielberger's Smoking Motivation Questionnaire', *Journal of Personality and Individual Differences*, vol. 14, pp. 629-37.

Pulver, A.E., Karayiorgou, M., Wolyniec, P.S., Lasseter, V.K., Wolyniec, P., Kasch, L., Antonarakis, S., Housman, D., Kazazian, H.H., Meyers, D., Nestadt, G., Ott, J., Liang, K.Y., Lamacz, M., Thomas, M., Childs, B., Diehl, S.R., Wang, S., Murphy, B., Sun, C.E. et al. (1994), 'Follow-up of a Report of a Potential Linkage for Schizophrenia on Chromosome 22 q12-q13.1: part 2', *American Journal of Medical Genetics*, vol. 54, pp. 44-50.

Pulver, A.E., Lassester, V.K., Kasch, L., et al. (1995), 'Schizophrenia: a genome scan targets chromosomes 3p and 8p as potential sites of susceptibility genes', *American Journal of Medical Genetics (Neuropsychiatric Genetics)*, vol. 60, pp. 252-60.

Quaid, K.A. (1994), 'A Few Words from a Wise Woman', in Weir, L., Fales, E. (eds), *Genes and Human Self-Knowledge*, pp. 77-8, University of Iowa Press, Iowa.

Ramsoy, N.R. (1966), 'Assortative Mating and the Structure of Cities', *American Sociological Review*, vol. 31, pp. 773-86.

Redlich, F. and Mollica, R.F. (1976) 'Overview: ethical issues in contemporary psychiatry', *American Journal of Psychiatry*, vol. 133, 125-36.

Reeder, S.T., Breuning, M.H., Davies, E., Nicolls, R.D., Jarman, A.P., Higgs, D.R., Pearson, P.L., Weatherall, D.J. (1985), 'A Highly Polymorphic DNA Marker Linked to Adult Polycystic Kidney Disease on Chromosome 16', *Nature*, vol. 317, pp. 542-5.

Reich, T. (1995), 'Genetic Linkage Studies of Bipolar Disorder', *Current Opinion in Psychiatry*, vol. 8, pp. 3-6.

Reik, T. (1957), *Of Love and Lust*, Jason Aronson, New York.

Reilly, P.R., Page, D.C. (1998), 'We're off to See the Genome', *Nature Genetics*, vol. 20, pp. 15-7.

Reiss, I.L. (1960), 'Toward a Sociology of the Heterosexual Love Relationship', *Marriage and Family Life*, vol. 22, pp. 139-45.

Reiss, I.L. (1965), 'Social Class and Campus Dating', *Social Problems*, vol. 13, pp. 193-204.

Reiss, I.L., Lee, G.R. (1988), F*amily Systems in America*, Holt, Rinehart and Winston, New York.

Reveley, A.M., Reveley, M.A., Murray, R.M. (1984), 'Cerebral Ventricular Enlargement in Non-genetic Schizophrenia: a controlled twin study', *British Journal of psychiatry*, vol. 144, pp. 89-93.

Reverley, A.M., Reverley, M.A., Clifford, C.A., Murray, R.M. (1982), 'Centrebral Ventricular size in twins discordant for schizophrenia', *Lancet*, vol. 6, pp. 540-1.

Richard, M.L., Liskow, B.I., Perry, P.J. (1985), 'Recent Psychostimulant Use in Hospitalized Schizophrenics', *Journal of Clinical Psychiatry*, vol. 39, pp. 425-6, 429-30.

Rinella, V.J. Jr., Gerstein, A.I. (1994), 'The Development of Dual Relationship: power and professional responsibility', *International Journal of Law and Psychiatry*, vol. 17, pp. 225-37.

Rogaev, E.I., Sherrington, R., Rogaeva, E.A., Levesqur, G., Ikeda, M., Liang, Y., Chi, H., Lin, C., Holman, K., Tsuda, T., Mar, L., Sorbi, S., Nacmias, B., Piacentini, S., Amaduccl, L., Chumakov, I., Cohen, D., Lannfelt, L., St. George-Hyslop, P.H. (1995), 'Familial Alzheimer's disease in Kindreds with Missense mutations in a Gene on Chromosome 1 Related to the Alzheimer's disease Type 3 Gene', *Nature*, vol. 376, pp. 775-9.

Roll-Hanssen, N. (1988), 'The Progress of Eugenics: growth of knowledge and change in ideology', *History of Science*, vol. 26, pp. 295-331.

Rosanoff, A.J., Handy, L.M., Plesset, I.R., Brush, S. (1934), 'The Etiology of So-called Schizophrenic Psychoses with Special Reference to Their Occurrence in Twins', *American Journal of Psychiatry*, vol. 91, pp. 247-86.

Rosenberg, M. (1965), *Society and The Adolescent Self-Image*, Princeton University Press, New Jersey.

Rosenthal, D, Kety, S.S. (eds.)(1968), *The Transmission of Schizophrenia*, Pergamon, Oxford.

Ross, C.A., McInnis, M.G., Margolis, R.L., Li, S.H. (1993), 'Genes with Triplet Repeats: candidate mediators of Neuropsychiatric Disorders', *Trends Neuroscience*, vol. 16, pp. 254-60.

Rubin, L.B. (1976), *Worlds of Pain: life in the working-class family*, Basic Books, New York.

Rubin, Z., Levinger, G. (1974), 'Theory and Data Badly Mated: a critique of Murstein's S.V.R. and Lewis's P.D.F. models of mate selection', *Journal of Marriage and the Family*, vol. 36, pp. 226-31.

Rutter, M., Plomin, R. (1997), 'Opportunities for Psychiatry from Genetic Findings', *British Journal of Psychiatry*, vol. 171, pp. 209-19.

Rychlak, J.F. (1965), 'The Similarity, Compatibility, or Incompatibility of Needs in Interpersonal Selection', *Journal of Personality and Social Psychology*, vol. 2, pp. 334-40.

Sadalla, E.K., Fausal, M. (1980), Dominance and Heterosexual Attraction: A Field Study, Unpublished manuscript, Arizona State University.

Sadalla, E.K., Kenrick, D.T., Vershure, B. (1987), 'Dominance and Heterosexual Attraction', *Journal of Personality and Social Psychology*, vol. 52, pp. 730-8.

Sasaki, T., Kennedy, J.L. (1995), 'Genetics of Psychosis', *Current Opinion in Psychiatry*, vol. 8, pp. 25-8.

Schafer, R.B., Keith, P.M. (1990), 'Matching by Weight in Married Couples: a life cycle perspective', *The Journal of Social Psychology*, vol. 130, No.5, pp. 657-64.

Schellenberg, J.A. (1960), 'Homogamy in Personal Values and the "Field of Eligibles"', *Social Forces*, vol. 39, pp. 157-62.

Schizophrenia Collaborative Linkage Group (Chromosome 22) (1996), 'A Combined Analysis of D22S278 Marker Alleles in Affected Sib-Pairs: Support for a Susceptibility Locus for Schizophrenia at Chromosome 22q12', *American Journal of Medical Genetics (Neuropsychiatric Genetics)*, vol. 67, pp. 40-5.

Schneier, F.R., Siris, S.G. (1987), 'A Review of Psychoactive Substance Use and Abuse in Schizophrenia: patterns of drug choice', *Journal of Nervous and Mental Disease*, vol. 175, pp. 641-52.

Schoen, R., Wooldredge, J. (1989), 'Marriage Choices in North Carolina and Virginia', *Journal of Marriage and The Family*, vol. 51, pp. 465-81.

Schuler, G.D., Boguski, M.S., Stewart, E.A. (1996), 'A Genetic Map of the Human Genome', *Science*, vol. 274, pp. 540-6.

Schulsinger, F., Parnas, J., Erling, T., Schulsinger, H., Teasdale, T.W., Mednick, S.A., Moller, L., Silverton, L. (1984), 'Cerebral Ventricular Size in the Offspring of Schizophrenic Mothers', *Archives of General Psychiatry*, vol. 44, pp. 602-6.

Schwab, S.G., Albus, M., Hallmayer, J., et al. (1995), 'Evaluation of a Susceptibility Gene for Schizophrenia on Chromosome 6p by Multipoint Affected Sib-Pair Linkage Analysis' *Nature Genetics*, vol. 11, pp. 325-7.

Scott, J.F. (1965), 'The American College Sorority: Its Role in Class and Ethnic Endogamy', *American Sociological Review*, vol. 30, pp. 514-27.

Seyfried, B.A. (1977), 'Complementarity in Interpersonal Attraction', in Duck, S.W. (ed.), *Theory and Practice in Interpersonal Attraction*, pp. 165-184, Academic Press, London.

Shepher, J., Reisman, J. (1985), 'Pornography: A Sociobiological Attempt at Understanding', *Ethology and Sociobiology*, vol. 6, pp. 103-14.

Sherrington, R., Rogaev, E.I., Liang, Y., et al. (1995), 'Cloning of a Gene Bearing Missense Mutations in Early Onset Familial Alzheimer's Disease', *Nature*, vol. 375, pp. 754-60.

Sherrington, R., Brynjolfsson, J., Petursson, H., Potter, M., Dudleston, K., Barraclough, B., Wasmuth, J., Dobbs, M., Gurling, H. (1988), 'Localization of a Susceptibility Locus for Schizophrenia on Chromosome 5', *Nature*, vol. 336, pp. 164-7.

Simpson, J.A., Kenrick, D.T. (1997), *Evolutionary Social Psychology*, Lawren Erlbaum, New Jersey.

Singh, D. (1993), Adaptive Significance of Female Physical Attractiveness: role of waist-to-hip ratio, Journal of Personality and Social Psychology, vol. 65, pp. 293-307.

Sipka, P., Lovre, M., Kosanovic, B., Kostic, P. (1988), 'Eksterna validacija skale L iz Eysenckovog testa licnosti EPQ. (External validity of the Eysenck Personality Questionnaire--Scale L.)', *Revija za Psihologiju*, vol. 18, pp. 9-17.

Slater, E. (1953), *Psychotic and Neurotic Illness in Twins*, MRC Special Publication 278, HMSO, London.

Slater, E., Woodside, M. (1951), *Patterns of Marriage*, Cassell, London.

Slobogin, C. (1996), 'Appreciation as a Measure of Competency: Some thoughts about the MacArthur Group's approach', *Psychology, Public Policy, and Law*, vol. 2, pp. 18-30.

Snell, R.G., Wilkins, R.J. (1986), 'Separation of Chromosomal DNA molecules from C.albicans by Pulsed Field Gel Electrophoresis', *Nucleic Acids Research*, vol. 14, pp. 4401-6.

Southern, E.M. (1975), 'Detection of Specific Sequences among DNA Fragments Separated by Gel Electrophoresis', *Journal of Molecular Biology*, vol. 98, pp. 502-3.

Spallone, P. (1989), Beyond Conception: the new politics of reproduction, MacMillan, London.

Spanier, G., Glick, P.C. (1980), 'Mate Selection Differentials between Whites and Blacks in the U.S.', *Social Forces*, vol. 58, pp. 707-25.

Spielberger, C.D. (1986), 'Psychological Determinants of Smoking Behavior', in Tollison, R.D. (ed.), *Smoking and Society: towards a more balanced assessment*, p89-134, D.C. Heath, Massachusetts.

St. George-Hyslop, P.H., Tanzi, R.E., Polinsky, R.J., Haines, R.J., Nee, L., Watkins, P.C., Myer, R.H., Feldman, R.G. (1987), 'The Genetic Defect Causing Familial Alzheimer's Disease Maps on Chromosome 21', *Science*, vol. 235, pp. 885-90.

Stefan, S. (1996), 'Race, Competence Testing, and Disability Law: a review of the MacArthur competence research', *Psychology, Public Policy, and Law*, vol. 2, pp. 31-44.

Stephen, T.D. (1984), 'A Symbolic Exchange Framework for the Development of Intimate Relationships', *Human Relations*, vol. 37, pp. 393-408.

Stephen, T.D. (1985), 'Fixed-Sequence and Circular-Casual Models of Relationship Development: Divergent Views on the Role of Communication in Intimacy', *Journal of Marriage and The Family*, vol. 47, pp. 955-63.

Stephen, T.D., Markman, H.J. (1983), 'Assessing the Development of Relationships: a new measure', *Family Process*, vol. 22, pp. 15-25.

Stevens, A., Price, J. (1996), *Evolutionary Psychiatry*, Routledge, London.

Straub, R., Lehner, T., Luo, Y., Loth, J.E., Shao, W., Sharpe, L., Alexander, J., Das, K., Simon, R., Fieve, R. et al. (1994), 'A Possible Vulnerability Locus for Bipolar Affective Disorder on Chromosome 21q22.3', *Nature Genetics*, vol. 8, pp. 291-6.

Surra, C.A. (1985), 'Courtship Types: variations in interdependence between partners and social networks', *Journal of Personality and Social Psychology*, vol. 56, pp. 357-75.

Surra, C.A. (1987), 'Reasons for Changes in Commitment: Variations by Courtship Style', *Journal of Social and Personal Relationships*, vol. 4, pp. 17-33.

Susanne, C., Lepage, Y. (1988), 'Assortative Mating for Anthropometric Characters', in Mascie-Taylor, C.G.N., Boyce, A.J. (eds.) *Human Mating Patterns*, Society for the Study of Human Biology Symposium 28, Cambridge University Press, Cambridge.

Svare, B., Kinsley, C.H. (1987), 'Hormones and Sex-Related Behavior: A Comparative Analysis', in Kelley, K. (ed.), *Females Men and Sexuality: theories and research*, pp. 13-58, State University of New York Press, Albany.

Szasz, T. (1986), 'Involuntary Mental Hospitalization: a crime against humanity', in Mappes, T.A. and Zembaty, J.S. (2nd edition), *Biomedical Ethics*, pp. 290-6, McGraw-Hill, New York.

Szasz, T. (1994a), *Cruel Compassion: psychiatric control of society's unwanted*, John Wiley and Son, New York.

Szasz, T. (1994b), 'Psychiatric Diagnosis, Psychiatric Power and Psychiatric Abuse', *Journal of Medical Ethics*, vol. 20, pp. 135-8.

Tarrier, N., Barraclough, C., Proceddu, K., Watts, S. (1988), 'The Assessment of Psychological Reactivity to the Expressed Emotion of the Relatives of Schizophrenic Patients', *British Journal of Psychiatry*, vol. 152, pp. 618-24.

Tharp, R.G. (1963), 'Psychological patterning in Marriage', *Psychological Bulletin*, vol. 60, pp. 97-117.

Thomasma, D.C. (1983), 'Limitations of the Autonomy Model for the Doctor-Patient Relationship. *Pharos*, vol. 46, pp. 2-5.

Tienari, P. (1975), 'Schizophrenia in Finnish Male Twins', in Lader, M.H. (ed.), *Studies of Schizophrenia*, pp. 29-35, Headley Brothers, Kent.

Trivers, R. (1985), *Social Evolution*, Benjamin / Cummings, California.

Tucker, M.B., Taylor, R.J. (1989), 'Demographic correlatives of Relationship Status among Black Americans', *Journal of Marriage and The Family*, vol. 51, pp. 655-65.

Uddenberg, N., Engelsson, Nettelbladt, P. (1979), 'Experience of Father and Later Relations to Men: A Systematic Study of Women's Relations to Their Father, Their Partner and Their Son', *Acta Psychiatrica Scandinavica*, vol. 59, pp. 87-96.

Vandenberg, S.G. (1972), 'Assortative Mating, or Who Marries Who?', *Behavior Genetics*, vol. 2, pp. 127-57.

Veatch, R.M. (1981), *A Theory of Medical Ethics*, Basic Books, New York.

Veatch, R.M., Flack, H.E. (1997), *Case Studies in Allied Health Ethics*, Prentice Hall, New Jersey.

Veevers, J.E. (1980), *Childless by Choice*, Butterworths, Toronto.

von der Lippe, A. L. (1965), 'Marital Partner Choice and Parental Identification', *Dissertation Abstracts*, vol. 26, No. 2.

von der Lippe, A. L. (1984), 'Parents and Partners: patterns of perceived similarity and their correlates in women', *Scandinavian Journal of Psychology*, vol. 25, pp. 348-62.

Wachs, T.D. (1993), 'The Nature-Nurture Gap: what we have here is a failure to collaborate', in Plomin, R., McClearn, G.E. (eds), *Nature Nurture and Psychology*, pp. 375-91.

Walster, E., Aronson, V., Abrahams, D., Rottmann, L. (1966), 'Importance of Physical Attractiveness in Dating Behavior', *Journal of Personality*, vol. 4, pp. 508-16.

Warner, R., Taylor, D., Wright, J., Sloat, A., Springett, G., Arnold, S., Weinberg, H. (1994), 'Substance Use among the Mentally Ill: prevalence, reasons for use, and effects on illness', *American Journal of Orthopsychiatry*, vol. 64, pp. 30-9.

Warren, M.A. (1997), *Moral Status – Obligations to Persons and Other Living Things*, Clarendon Press, Oxford.

Watkins, M.P., Meredith, W. (1981), 'Spouse Similarity in Newlyweds with Respect to Specific Cognitive Abilities, Socioeconomic Status, and Education', *Behavior Genetics*, vol. 11, pp. 1-21.

Watson, C.G., Kucala, T., Tilleskjor, C., Jacobs, L. (1984a), 'Schizophrenic Birth Seasonality in Relation to the Incidence of Infectious Disease and Temperature Extremes', *Archives of General Psychiatry*, vol. 41, pp. 85-90.

Watson, C.G., Tilleskjor, C., Pucell, J., Jacobs, L. (1984b), 'Do Alcoholics Give Valid Self-Report?' *Journal of Studies on Alcohol*, vol. 45, pp. 344-8.

Weinstock, R., Leong, G.B. (1996), 'Ethical Issues in Psychiatry', *Current Opinion in Psychiatry*, vol. 9, pp. 407-11.

Weissman, M.M., Gershon, E.S., Kidd, K.K. (1984), 'Psychiatric Disorders in the Relatives of Probands with Affective Disorder', *Archives of General Psychiatry*, vol. 41, pp. 13-21.

Welsh, M.J., Tsui, L.C., Boat, J.F., Beauder, A.L. (1995), 'Cystic Fibrosis', in Scriver, C.R., Beaudet, A.L., Sly, W.S., Valle, D. (eds.), *The Metabolic and Molecular Bases of Inherited Disease*, pp. 3799-876, McGraw-Hill, New York.

Wexler, N. (1992), 'Clairvoyance and Caution: repercussions from the Human Genome Project', in Kelves, D.J., Hood, L. (eds.), *The Code of Codes: scientific and social issues in the Human Genome Project*, pp. 221-43, Harvard University Press, London.

White, R., Leppert, D., Bishop, T., Barker, D., Berkowitz, J., Brown, C., Callahan, P., Holm, T. (1985), 'Construction of Linkage Maps with DNA Markers for Human Chromosomes', *Nature*, vol. 313, pp. 101-5.

Williams, T. (1975), 'Family resemblance in abilities: the Weschsler Scales', *Behavioral Genetics*, vol. 5, pp. 405-9.

Wilson, D.J., Doolabh, A. (1992), 'Reliability, factorial validity and equivalence of several forms of the Eysenck Personality Inventory/ Questionnaire in Zimbabwe', *Personality and Individual Differences*, vol. 13, pp. 637-43.

Wilson, W.J. (1987), *The Truly Disadvantaged*, University of Chicago Press, Chicago.

Winch, R.F. (1955a), 'The Theory of Complementary Needs in Mate Selection: A Test of One Kind of Complementariness', *American Sociological Review*, vol. 20, pp. 52-6.

Winch, R.F. (1955b), 'The Theory of Complementary Needs in Mate Selection: final results on the test of the general hypothesis', *American Sociological Review*, vol. 20, pp. 552-5.

Winch, R.F. (1958), *Mate Selection: a study of complementary needs*, Harper, New York.

Winch, R.F., Ktsanes, T., Ktsanes, V. (1955), 'Empirical Elaboration of the Theory of Complementary Needs in Mate Selection', *Journal of Abnormal and Social Psychology*, vol. 51, pp. 508-13.

Winick, B.J. (1996), 'Foreward: a summary of the MacArthur Treatment Competence Study and an Introduction to the Special Theme', *Psychology, Public Policy, and Law*, vol. 2, pp. 3-17.

Wolfe, D.M. (1959), 'Power and Authority in the Family' , in Cartwright, D. (ed.), *Studies in Social Power*, pp. 99-117, Institute for Social Research, Ann Arbor, Michigan.

Wragg, M., Hutton, M., Talbot, C. (1996), 'Genetic Association between Intronic Polymorphism in Presenilin-1 Gene and Late-Onset Alzheimer's Disease', *Lancet*, vol. 347, pp. 509-12.

Yates, J.R.W., Conner, J.M. (1986), 'Genetic Linkage', *British Journal of Hospital Medicine*, vol. 36, pp. 133-6.

Zeiss, R.A., Tanke, E.D., Fenn, H.H., Yesavage, J.A. (1996), 'Dangerousness Commitments: indices of future violence potential?', *Bulletin of American Academy of Psychiatry and Law*, vol. 24, pp. 247-53.

Index

For Product Safety Concerns and Information please contact our EU
representative GPSR@taylorandfrancis.com
Taylor & Francis Verlag GmbH, Kaufingerstraße 24, 80331 München, Germany

www.ingramcontent.com/pod-product-compliance
Ingram Content Group UK Ltd.
Pitfield, Milton Keynes, MK11 3LW, UK
UKHW022202190926
475702UK00003B/159
* 9 7 8 1 1 3 8 3 4 7 8 9 2 *